T0042213

Dr. Kellon's Guide To

FIRST AID FOR HORSES

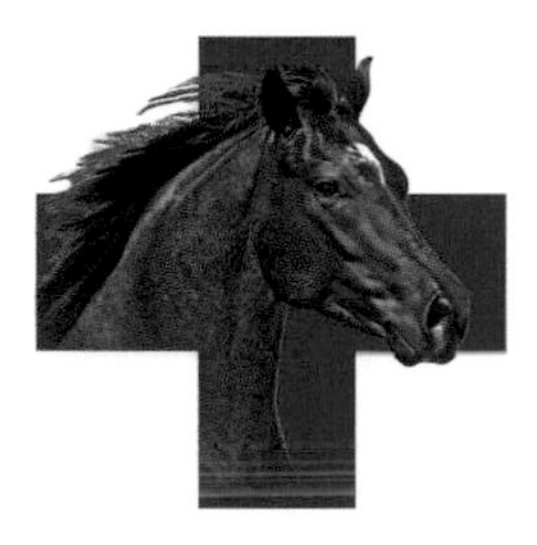

Eleanor Kellon, VMD

Includes special sections on emergency splinting techniques by the Center for Equine Health, UC Davis School of Veterinary Medicine, and on trailer accidents and other emergencies by Dr. Rebecca Gimenez, a primary instructor in Technical Large Animal Emergency Rescue.

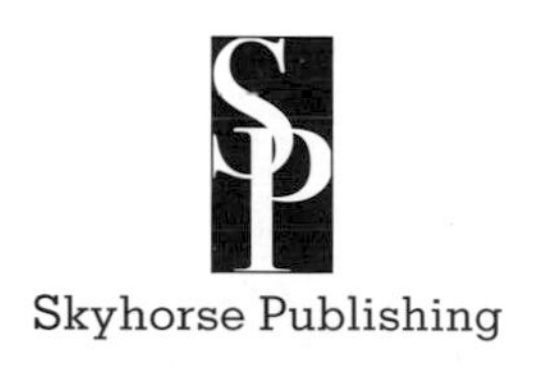

Skyhorse Publishing books may be purchased in bulk at special discounts for sales promotion, corporate gifts, fund-raising, or educational purposes. Special editions can also be created to specifications. For details, contact the Special Sales Department, Skyhorse Publishing, 307 West 36th Street, 11th Floor, New York, NY 10018 or info@skyhorsepublishing.com.

Visit our website at www.skyhorsepublishing.com.

10 9 8 7 6

Library of Congress Cataloging-in-Publication Data is available on file.

Cover design by Tom Lau
Cover image credit: iStockphoto.com
Interior photo credits: Donna Brown, Larry Catt, Candace Craw-Goldman, Donna Dixon-Woodall, Maureen Gallatin, Rebecca Gimenez, Charles Hilton, Fran Jurga, Nancy Kerns, Isabel Kurek, Diane Nicholson, Becky Siler, Sue Stuska, and Stefan Witte

Print ISBN: 978-1-5107-4166-9
Ebook ISBN: 978-1-5107-4168-3

Printed in China

A MESSAGE FROM THE AUTHOR AND THE PUBLISHER

This book is not intended to be used as a substitute for veterinary care, or as a "do-it-yourself" manual. The situations covered are genuine emergencies (with the exception of some entries that the owner or other caretaker might confuse for an emergency) and therefore warrant veterinary care. In some instances, guidelines have been given on how long it would be acceptable to wait before having the veterinarian see the horse. However, this is based strictly on average, uncomplicated cases and should not be used as a hard and fast rule.

The veterinarian should be contacted as soon as possible if any of the problems described herein are encountered. It is always important to clear any recommended procedures or medications with the veterinarian prior to implementing them.

Horses vary significantly in their reactions to stress and medications, so any dosages, procedures or recommendations are strictly based on generally accepted averages and are not intended as specific instructions for any individual horse.

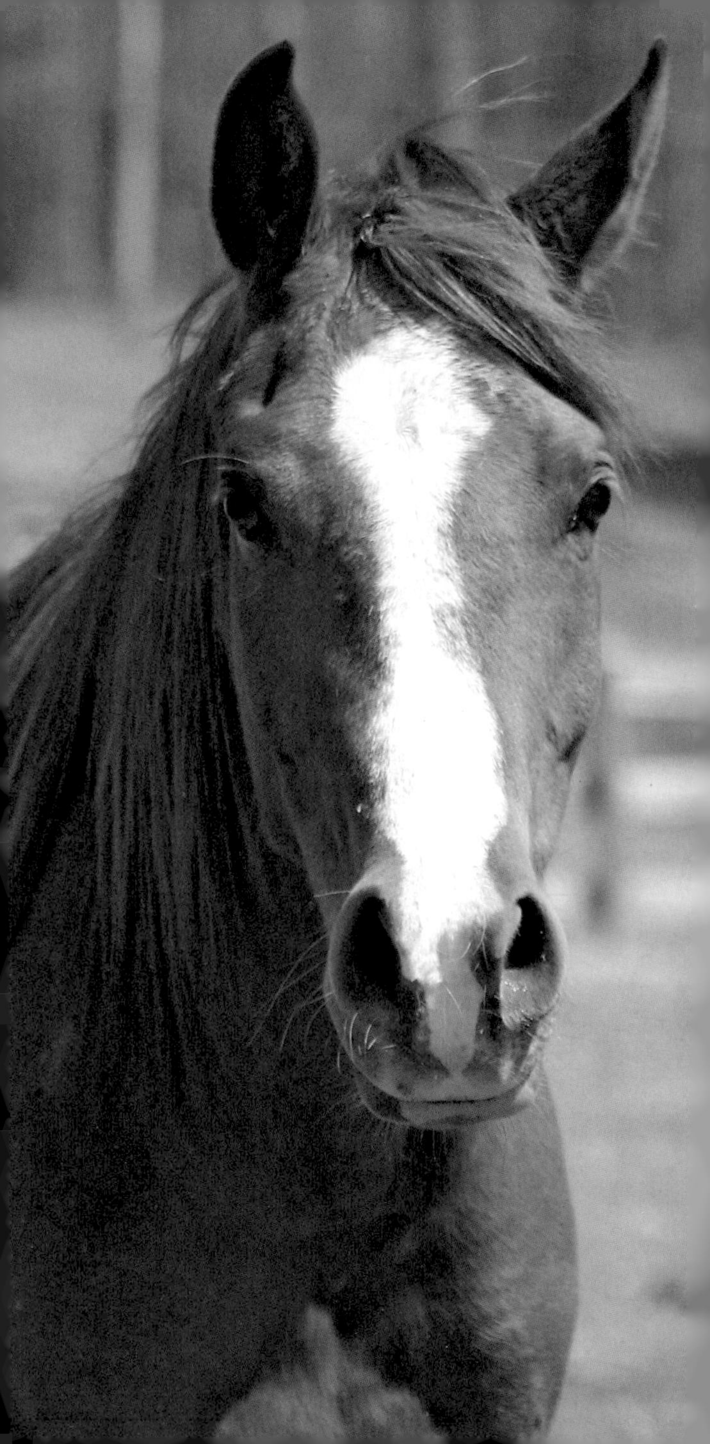

CONTENTS

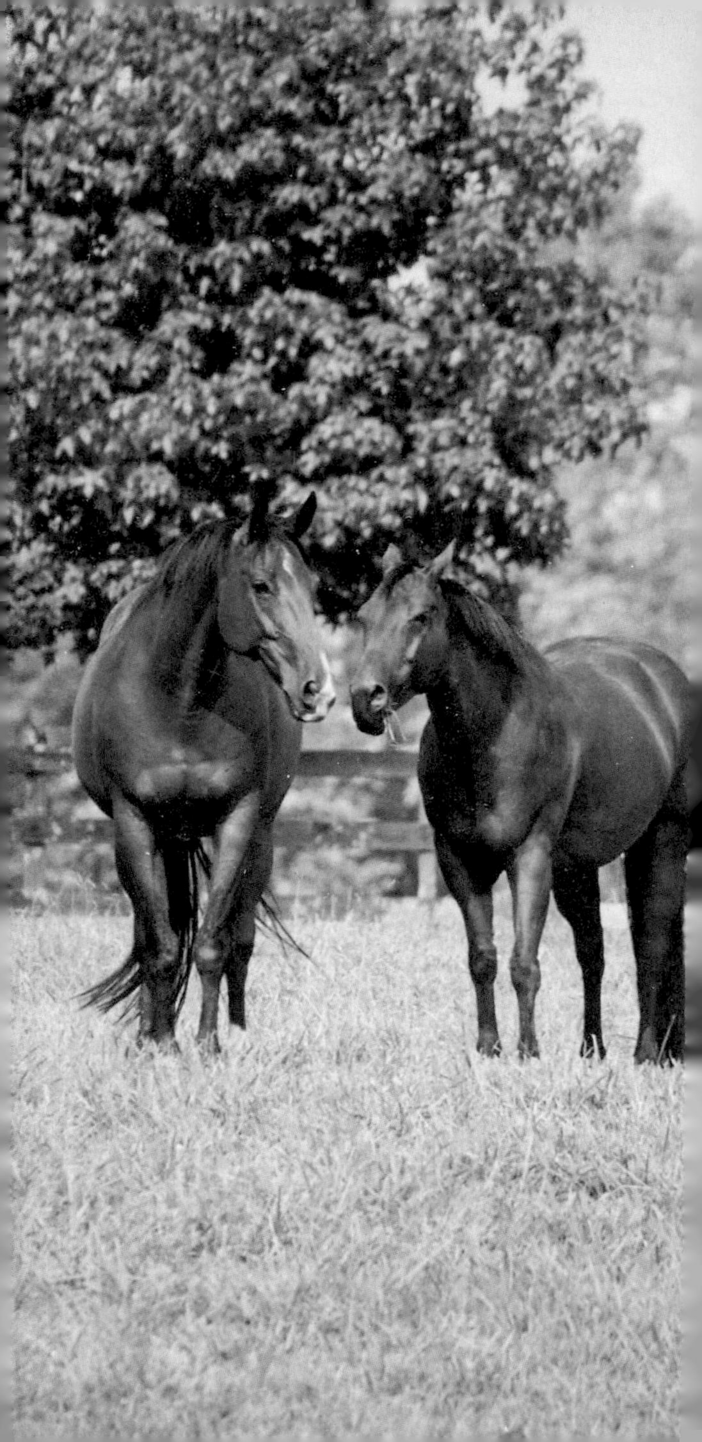

01
GUIDELINES

2

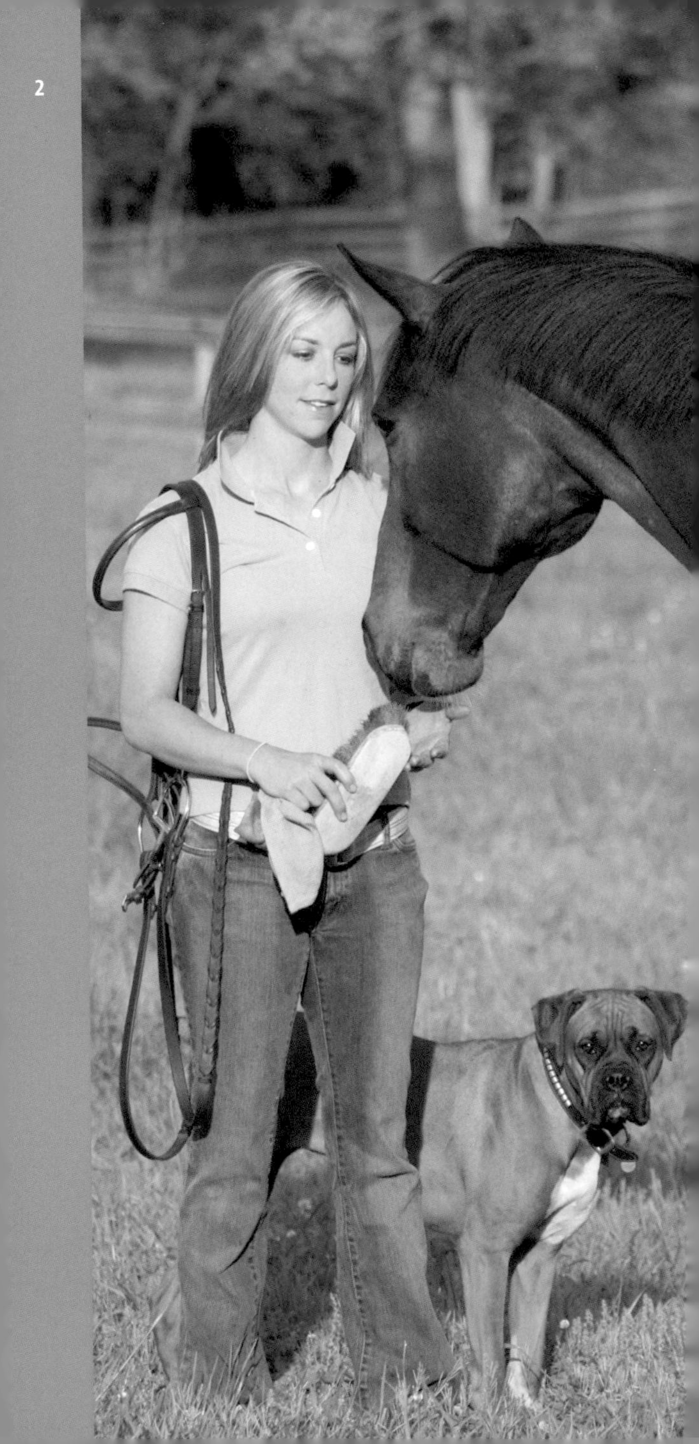

GUIDELINES

The purpose of this book is to provide quick and easy reference to conditions that require emergency treatment and to advise what you can do until the veterinarian arrives. It is not intended to replace diagnosis and treatment by your veterinarian. However, it offers guidelines to be followed in determining what a horse's problem could be, and it suggests information that should be given to the veterinarian as soon as you call.

This book is organized by chapters on specific types of problems (e.g., Wounds, Bleeding, Burns, etc.) or on specific anatomical areas (e.g., Eyes) and organ systems (e.g. Disorders of Eating and Colic). At the beginning of each chapter is a quick reference list of symptoms and topics that allows you to turn immediately to those sections of the chapter that might pertain to your horse's problems.

If you are unsure about what organ system your horse's symptoms are related to, turn to the complete index at the end of the book. This will also refer you to any other organ system that you may not have realized may be involved in the problem. For example, "salivation" ("drooling," "foaming at the mouth") will refer you to the chapter on Disorders of Eating, as well as to the chapters on Collapse/Seizures and Disorders of Balance (Botulism and Rabies).

The sections are also keyed by a system of block icons as follows:

■ Serious illness, get attention within 24 hours;
■■ Requires veterinary attention that day;
■■■ Potentially life-threatening, seek immediate veterinary attention.

You'll also see an ℞ beside many drug names. Drugs with this icon must be obtained from your vet or purchased using a prescription supplied by your vet. Even if you have these items on hand, they should NEVER be used without consulting with your vet first. Never use human medications or over-the-counter drugs such as penicillin, tetanus toxoid or tetanus antitoxin, without your vet's approval, either. We've listed some of these medications on the First Aid Kit pages because they'll be referenced in the chapter that follows, but that does not mean they should be kept on hand. Also remember that some drugs must be kept refrigerated, and all have expiration dates.

Chapter 24 provides reference material and other information that should be helpful for you in emergency situations. Chapter 25 contains how-to-instructions for many common procedures, such as taking a horse's pulse. Chapter 26 details emergency splinting techniques, and Chapter 27 contains guidelines for handling trailer accidents or other horse-related emergencies. Should you encounter a word that you don't recognize, consult the Glossary on page 322.

Finally, we recommend that you take a few minutes to fill in the important numbers on the last page of this book, so you'll have them handy in case of emergency.

Dr. Kellon's Guide To

FIRST AID FOR HORSES

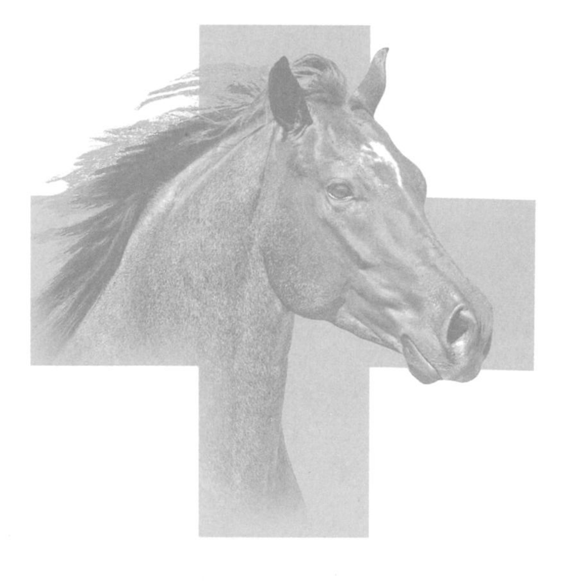

02

PREPARATION AND VITAL SIGNS

BE PREPARED

Perhaps you've wondered how you might handle an emergency situation with horses, should you have to. In fact, the people who perform best under emergency situations are those who know what to do. Advance preparation, good organization and a cool head are all needed.

We recommend that you become familiar with this book before you actually need it. This will make it easier for you to find the information you need quickly, and may prevent your making a mistake if the book is not at hand the moment you need it. (For example, you might remember from your reading that it is potentially harmful to force a horse that is tying up to walk.)

Advance preparation should also include assembling your first aid supplies and filling in emergency phone numbers.

VITAL INFO

In addition to providing emergency first aid before the vet arrives, you should assemble vital information necessary to make a diagnosis (The Information sheet in the Appendix, page 325 will be helpful for this.) You'll want to have this data on hand when you call the vet, although in certain situations, as when a horse is experiencing heavy arterial bleeding, basic information (such as, "My horse is bleeding from an artery in his left leg, is lying flat on the ground and trembling") will provide the vet with enough information to be able to tell you what to do next.

Here's the info you should note:

- Pulse and respiration rates
- Temperature (rectal)
- Mucous membrane color
- Posture (limping, head hanging, etc.)
- Behavior — note anything abnormal
- Your general impression about the horse
- Condition of the stall, bedding, manure, etc.
- Any possible causes or recent changes that may factor in, such as feed, bedding, medications, etc.

PULSE AND RESPIRATION RATES

When a horse is in pain, the release of stress hormones causes him to breathe more rapidly and his heart to beat faster than normal.

A normal pulse rate is anywhere from the high 20s to the low 40s (beats per minute), depending on how excited the horse is at the time, as well as the weather and his level of fitness.

NORMAL VALUES FOR A HORSE AT REST — TPR (Temperature, Pulse, and Respiration)

Temperature:	98°F to 100°F
Pulse:	44 beats per minute (Range high 20s to low 40s)
Respiration:	8 to 16 breaths per minute

Weather conditions will affect values (i.e., higher on hot days). Excitement and fear will quickly elevate pulse and respiration, which will just as quickly return to normal when the animal is quiet. Foals will tend to run in the upper ranges.

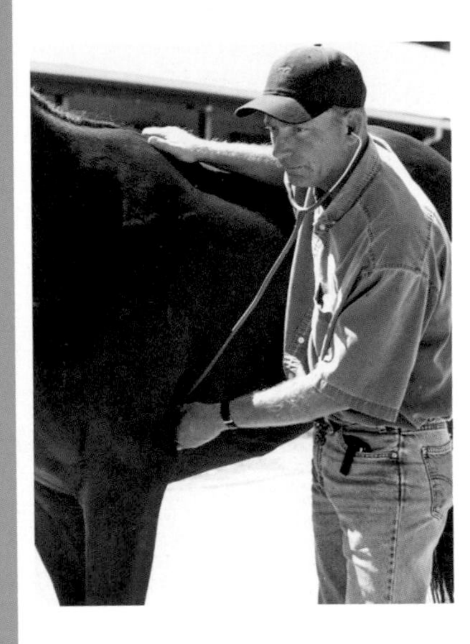

To obtain a heart rate without feeling for a pulse, listen to the heart with a stethoscope slid under the horse's left elbow.

You can check a horse's pulse at several locations, the easiest being under the jaw — the pulse in the facial artery. (See Chapter 25, page 253)

A respiratory rate is obtained simply by counting how many times the horse's chest moves in and out over a minute. Each in-and-out is counted as one breath. Be sure to count for a full minute, rather than 15 seconds multiplied by four, since horses normally breathe as slowly as 8 breaths per minute.

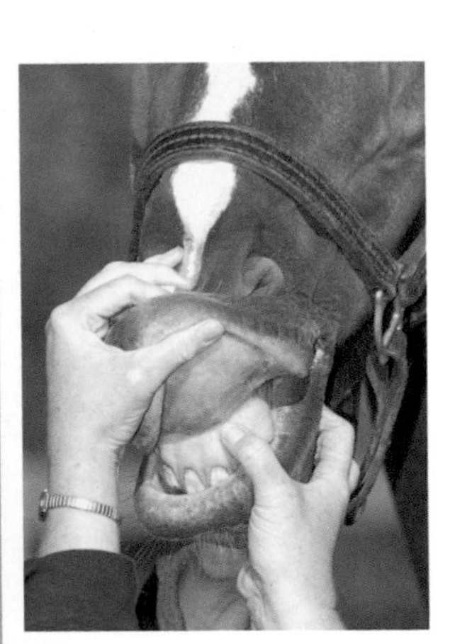

To determine the capillary refill time, gently press your finger against the horse's gum, then withdraw it. Count how long it takes for the gum color to return.

TEMPERATURE

High body temperatures occur when the horse has been struggling, or with infections. Lower-than-normal temperatures can be seen with shock or life-threatening infections, especially in foals. Extremes of overheating or cold weather may also cause above-or below-normal body temperature

The horse's temperature is taken rectally. See Chapter 25, page 253.

MUCOUS MEMBRANE COLOR

The color of the mucous membranes, such as the gums, provides important clues to the horse's overall condition:

- Very pale or white indicates blood loss, early shock or severe pain.
- Bright red indicates a toxic condition or exertion.
- Gray-blue indicates severe shock.

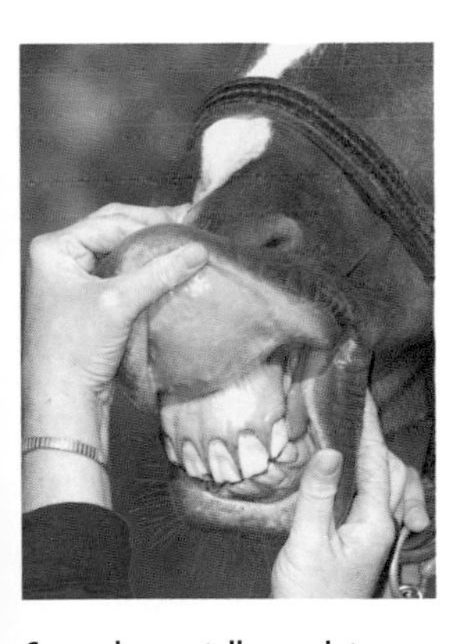

Gum color can tell you a lot about the horse's condition. Take a moment to notice what's normal for your healthy horse.

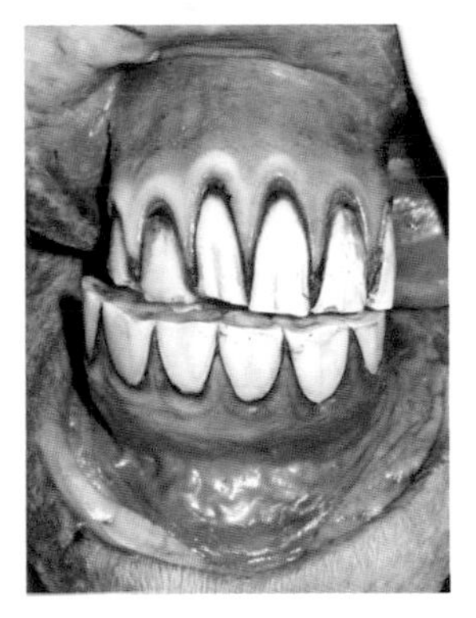

Horses severely toxic from bacteria toxins have blue to purplish gums.

- Bright yellow indicates possible liver disease.

Applying light pressure with your fingertips to the mucous membranes can reveal clues to the horse's health. Light pressure causes the mucous membranes to blanch. The amount of time it takes the color to return after the pressure is released (usually around one to two seconds) is called the "capillary refill time." In a shock-like state with dehydration, the capillary refill time is prolonged.

You can practice this technique on your own finger or toenails. The pressure needed to result in a white spot is the same pressure to apply to a horse's gums.

OTHER OBSERVATIONS

- Make note of anything abnormal about the horse's behavior and appearance. The information may be specific — such as the refusal to open an eye and tearing — or, more general — such as depression, trembling, or sweating. Everything you note could be important.
- Check the feed bin, water bucket and hay supply. Observe the stall or corral for the character and quantity of urine and feces. Observe the bedding for any signs of thrashing or struggling around.
- If you know when the horse first became ill or injured, record this. If not, note when he was last seen well and when he was found ill.
- After the veterinarian has been called, continue with the recommended emergency treatments or those ordered by your vet. While waiting for the vet to arrive, you should record the TPR (temperature, pulse, and respiration) at 15- to 20-minute intervals in life-threatening situations. Also check the mucous membranes and note any changes in symptoms.

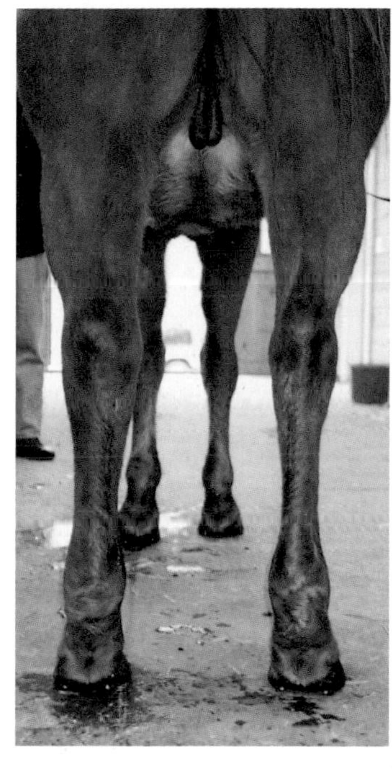
Swelling in one leg only isn't likely to be simple stocking up. It may be caused by infection, injury or old damage to the circulation or lymphatic system.

- Finally, when you have a minute, try to think of anything that might have caused or contributed to the problem, or of any similar episodes in the past. Write them down so you don't forget to mention them in the commotion after the veterinarian arrives. Never rely on your memory during an emergency. There is simply too much going on to remember all these pieces of information.

As for keeping a cool head, nothing will calm you quicker than having something to do and getting on with it. Company helps too, so phone for nearby help as soon as you make contact with the vet. Do not hesitate to enlist the help of paramedics, the fire department or similar services if the animal is trapped. They may not be familiar with horses, but they will know how best to free a trapped horse and can assist you with basic first aid techniques.

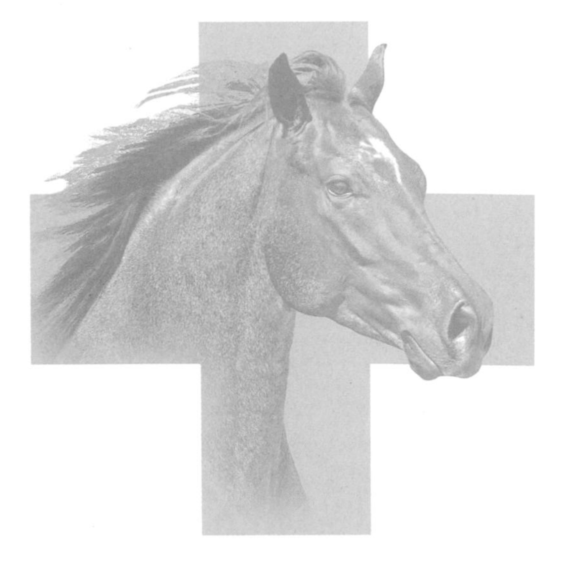

03

RESTRAINT OF THE ILL OR INJURED HORSE

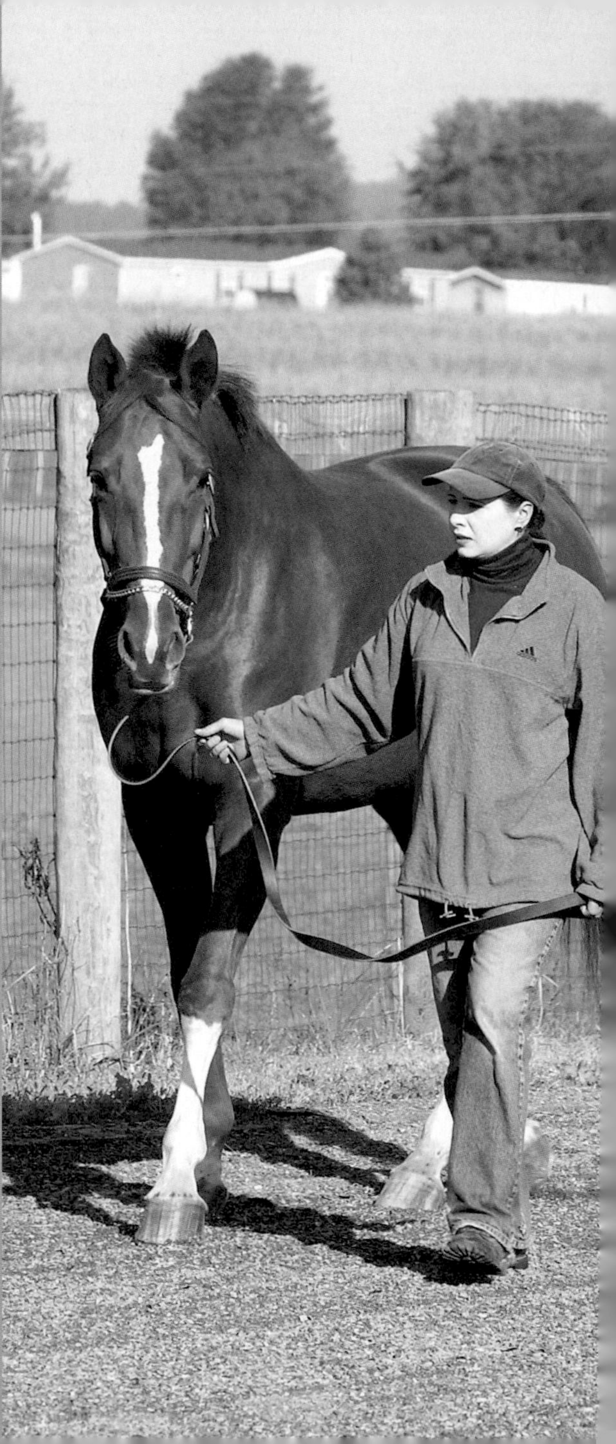

RESTRAINT OF THE ILL OR INJURED HORSE

Before initiating any emergency treatment or even examining the horse, it is necessary to assess the horse's state of mind and establish adequate restraint. Horses vary in their response to pain and frightening circumstances. For example, a trapped horse — whether entangled in barbed wire, stuck in a trailer accident, or simply cast in his stall — may struggle wildly or he may lie perfectly still, as if in a trance.

A frantic horse is dangerous to himself and anyone who attempts to approach him. Before approaching the animal, be certain you have his attention. Keeping a safe distance, locate yourself close to his head (not his tail) and speak to him softly. Continue to make attempts to get the horse's attention by speaking softly. This will often calm the horse enough for you to approach. If the horse will not quiet down or he seems totally unaware of your presence, don't attempt to go closer until you have help. The horse that seems calm, perhaps even too calm under the circumstances, may be in shock or afraid that any move he makes will cause pain. Such a horse must also be handled carefully, as he may explode at any moment.

For example, I recall a carriage horse that was tied to a hitching post out of sight. Suddenly a loud crash was heard, and the horse was found lying flat on the ground. Her breathing was very slow and regular, her pulse normal. Only her eyes were moving. Help was assembled and the harness loosened. As the carriage was being pulled back, the horse suddenly began lurching violently and threw herself forward, only to collapse again. It was immediately obvious that she had somehow managed to impale herself on one of the shafts, which had been driven into her underarm and along the chest wall for a distance of approximately eight inches. This horse knew, as many do, that struggling under the circumstances could easily have injured her further. However, the minute she was released (and/or when she felt the pain of the shaft being removed), the instinct to flee became overwhelming.

This same mare is a good example of how a horse in shock should be handled. After the initial release, the mare was trembling badly and very shaky on her feet. Her gums were extremely white, and she was indifferent to the people and things around her, also refusing to eat or drink. There was initial concern she might be bleeding internally, but her strong and steady pulse argued against this. The horse was in a state of shock, triggered by her severe injury.

During this time, it was possible to carefully examine, probe, clean and flush her wound with no restraint other than a lead shank. She showed virtually no reaction to the injection of local anesthesia prior to suturing the wound. However, after general supportive measures of blanketing the mare and administering a dose of phenylbutazone to ease her pain, the situation became quite different, and she violently resisted any attempt to even approach the area of the injury. She was a very large mare and quite used to having her own way, so it was necessary to use a twitch for the next three days of treatments. After that time, the pain had eased enough that treatments could again be managed with only a lead shank.

METHODS OF RESTRAINT

If the horse needs restraint, choose a method that will give you the most effective control in that situation. Restraint methods used properly will stop the horse from fighting the handler. "Properly" is the catch, and the reason that many vets prefer to use their own handler when dealing with difficult restraint situations. It's a judgment call, however, as the safety of the people involved and the need to administer emergency treatments must remain paramount.

The simplest method of restraint is the **lead rope** or **lead shank**, simply clipped to the bottom ring of the halter. Basically, this lets the handler keep the horse from moving around and allows the handler to manipulate him in any direction desired. The handler should stand just in front of the horse's shoulder, never directly in front of the horse (lest the horse strike) and on the same side as the veterinarian or person treating or examining the horse. Should the horse act up, in most cases the handler can pull the horse's head toward himself. That will prevent the horse from moving his hind end into the handler or examiner, or from kicking them with his hind feet.

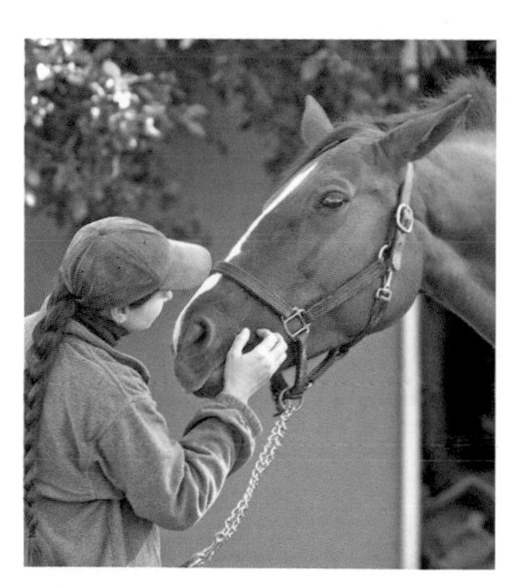

A simple lead rope and a few kind words may calm or distract a horse under normal conditions, but most first-situations will require additional restraint.

Another effective method of restraint is **picking up a horse's leg**. This is usually done when a horse has a limb problem and keeps lifting his leg or kicking when being treated. When working on the hind end, pick up the front leg on the same side as the one being treated. When working on the forequarters, pick up the opposite front leg. One drawback of this maneuver is the very real possibility that the horse will continue to struggle and, being off balance, may actually fall. It's not recommended for high-strung horses, but is most useful for those that fidget or lift a leg automatically every time it is touched.

The **twitch** is an effective device for achieving control. It's been documented that a horse's heart rate actually drops when he's twitched — an indication that the horse is both calmer and not feeling pain from the twitch. Several types of twitches are available, including short and long-handled twitches with rope or chain on the end, and smooth metal twitches that are self-retaining and attach to the halter. The advantage of hand-held twitches is that they can be tightened or loosened as needed during the treatment. However, even the less severe self-retaining twitches work well under most circumstances and can be squeezed tighter by hand if need be. (See Chapter 25, page 256 for how to apply a twitch.)

When using a twitch, the most resistance is usually encountered during the procedure of trying to apply it. Once in place, the horse may attempt to back, rear or toss his head to get free. However, after the initial resistance, most horses will stand quietly for routine treatments when twitched. The effectiveness of this device seems to transcend the actual discomfort it may cause. Some horses appear to doze while twitched. In any event, do not hesitate to use this effective method to facilitate treatments.

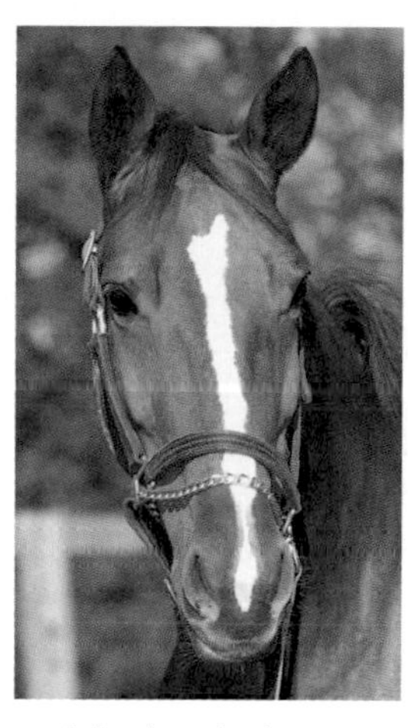

When using a chain over the nose, a few quick, light jerks are more effective in getting the horse's attention than using extended pressure.

A variation of the simple lead is a **chain lead shank**, with the chain run over the nose or under the jaw. This works well for horses that fidget or try to avoid treatment but don't require twitching. When held quietly, the chain doesn't bother the horse. However, should more restraint be needed, a few quick jerks will get the horse's attention. Be aware that activating the effect of the chain may make the horse back up or raise his head. If you get this reaction, wait a few seconds for the horse to settle. Adjust tension on the chain so there is just enough to remind the horse that the chain is there, and proceed. If the horse resists again, use a twitch or position the chain in the horse's mouth.

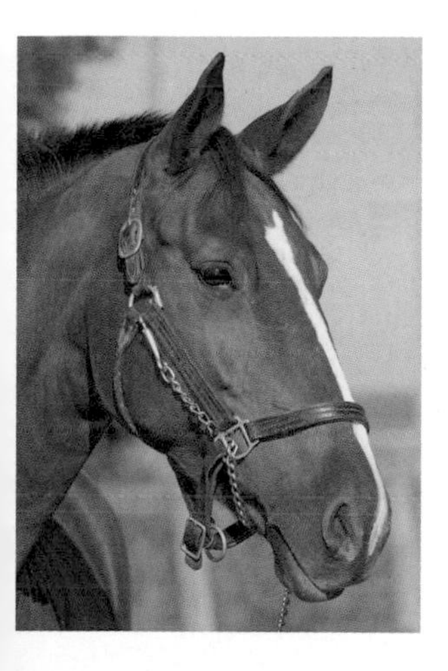

A lead chain can be **passed through the mouth** like a bit and hooked to the halter ring on the opposite side. It is effective without actually injuring the

Using a chain under the horse's chin will often cause the horse to raise his head and sometimes to rear or attempt to pull away.

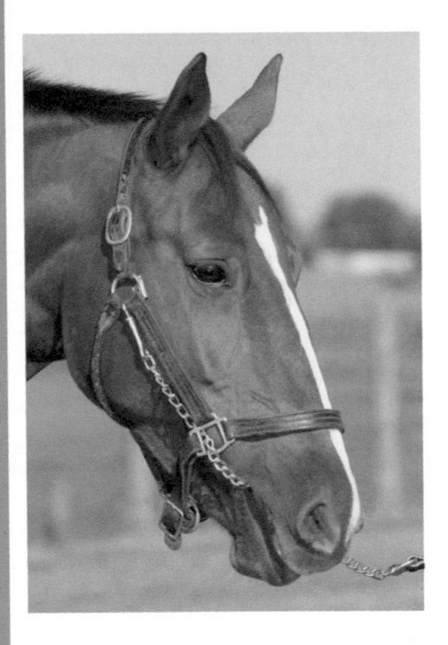

When using a chain through the horse's mouth, clip it to the top ring of the halter, rather than to the noseband ring.

horse. It's most effectively used when the handler gives a few small jerks to get the horse's attention prior to the start of treatments and then keeps a light tension on the shank until the horse is resigned to being treated. Most horses will respect this almost as much as a twitch, though a twitch should always be tried before resorting to a chain through the mouth.

A more severe use of the chain shank, usually reserved for horses that cannot be twitched and for some reason should not be tranquilized, is running a chain on the gum, **under the upper lip**. Chains placed on the sensitive gums can cause significant pain and even bleeding if the horse fights it (as many will do). However, once the initial fight is over, the degree of restraint is equivalent to twitching, provided slight tension is kept on the chain. If allowed to go slack, it may slip off and into the mouth. Repositioning it is likely to cause additional anxiety.

The use of chains for restraint should only be done by people experienced with this technique. When used too vigorously or not convincingly enough, the horse is likely to fight.

Finally, there are **tranquilizers** — chemical restraint. Tranquilizers do not replace physical restraint, nor do they eliminate the possibility the horse will resist treatment. However, they do slow the horse's responses, calm anxiety and today's combinations often help with pain. Pain will still generate a response, and even a tranquilized horse is quite capable of inflicting serious injury. Tranquilizers should only be administered by, or on the direction of, a vet.

For most non-veterinarians, the intramuscular route is preferable to the intravenous route, since accidental injection of some tranquilizers into an artery rather than a vein can cause severe reactions. This is a very real possibility with injections made high in the neck, where the needle may be injected at the wrong angle and penetrate an artery. With intramuscular injections, allow 15 to 20 minutes for the tranquilizer to take effect. See Chapter 23, page 205 for signs of adequate tranquilization.

Do not use tranquilizers with horses that:

- Have sustained a significant blood loss.
- Appear to be in shock.
- May have extensive internal injuries.
- May have a disturbed fluid balance (such as with colic, heat stroke, or urinary tract problems).

When properly used, tranquilizers are often a valuable adjunct to handling a fractious horse. By alleviating anxiety, they make the treatment process safer for both horse and handlers. Beyond the first-aid situation, the use of tranquilizers can often be discontinued once the horse learns the routine of the treatment and what to expect and/or when the condition being treated is not as painful as in the acute stages.

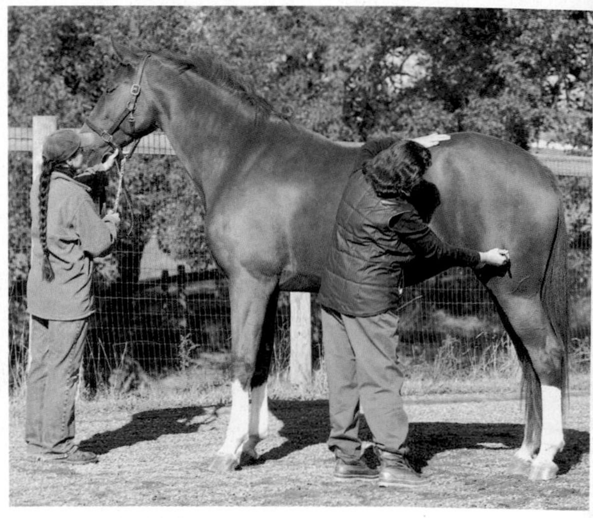

Generally speaking, when the vet is examining or treating the horse, the handler should stand on the same side of the horse as the vet.

SUMMARY

- Proper assessment of the horse's state of mind, while unpredictable, is essential to achieving control.
- Once you have his attention and have made contact, restraint should be appropriate to the degree of resistance the horse shows.
- The depressed, "shocky" horse does not need to be twitched in most cases. In fact, to do so is an unnecessary stress to the already over-stressed animal.
- The horse that actively resists treatment will need effective restraint for his own good and the safety of all.
- Choose the least aggressive method that will still adequately restrain the horse.
- Tranquilizers should only be administered on the advice of a veterinarian.

04 WOUNDS

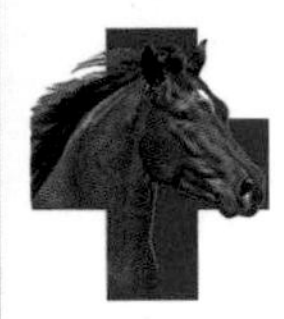

FIRST AID KIT

- Iodine-based surgical scrub (soap) or hexachlorophene soap
- Antibiotic ointment
- Iodine ointment
- Sterile gauze pads
- Wound spray
- Scarlet Red
- Blukote
- Alushield
- Tetanus toxoid ℞
- Tetanus antitoxin ℞
- Quilted cotton leg bandages
- Cloth or self-adhesive leg wraps, such as Vetrap™
- Antibiotics ℞
  - — Injectable (Penicillin—no steroids)
  - — Oral (Trimethoprim-sulfadiazine tablets)
- Phenylbutazone
- ℞ Blanket
- Epsom salts

℞: PRESCRIPTION DRUG — MUST BE OBTAINED FROM VETERINARIAN OR PRESCRIBED BY A VET — SHOULD NEVER BE ADMINISTERED WITHOUT PRIOR APPROVAL BY A VETERINARIAN.

QUICK CHAPTER REFERENCE LIST

LEGEND: ■■■ — NEEDS EMERGENCY ATTENTION; ■■ — SHOULD BE EXAMINED BY A VET;
■ — MAY NEED VETERINARY ADVICE/ATTENTION

WOUNDS

When dealing with wounds of any kind, your primary concerns are to stop any bleeding and clean the wound of foreign debris.

SUPERFICIAL WOUNDS ■

Definition: *Superficial wounds involve loss of hair and minimal skin penetration.*

Abrasions and lacerations

Abrasions are brush-burn-type injuries (such as rope burns) with loss of hair and minimal loss of skin, usually accompanied by oozing of clear fluids (serum) and some slow ooze of blood.

Lacerations penetrate the skin. With superficial lacerations, only the upper layers of skin are damaged. Typically, the edges of the wound will remain close together. There may be more bleeding than with abrasions, but this is easily controlled by pressure, or it stops on its own within minutes.

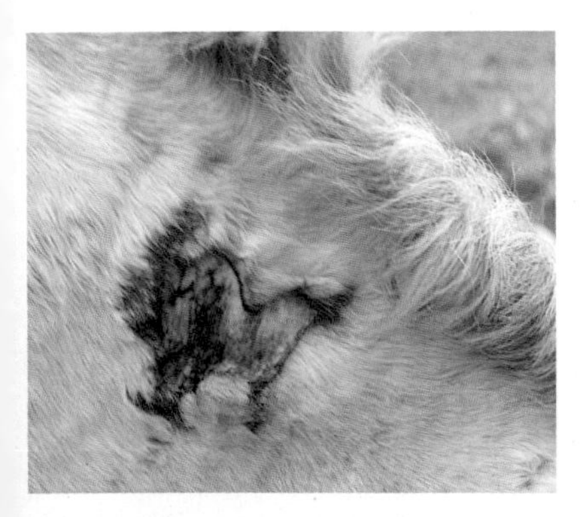

This skin laceration will heal very well with suturing since there's no actual damage to the tissue underneath.

Treatment:

- Hose the area with cool water for 10 minutes.
- Follow this by gentle cleaning, using gauze and Betadine surgical scrub or a hexachlorophene soap (e.g., pHisoDerm). If these aren't available, use any gentle soap, such as Ivory. Begin cleaning at the top of the wound and work down. (The horse may need restraint in addition to a lead rope or crossties.)
- Do not use cotton balls or cotton when cleaning wounds, as the lint fibers may cause contamination.
- Rinse well and inspect for any remaining debris or dirt.
- Allow the area to dry, then apply antibiotic ointment or iodine ointment to the wound.
- Apply a sterile gauze or Telfa pad over the wound and secure it in place with either a partial bandage of the self-adhering type (e.g., Vetrap) or a standard leg bandage. Injuries located on areas that cannot be bandaged should be dressed with the antibiotic ointment, as above, and repeatedly checked for any accumulating dirt, straw, etc., then re-cleaned and ointment reapplied as necessary. Keep flies away from the wound area.

As an alternative treatment, Scarlet Red, Blukote, Alushield or any similar wound spray may be used and is less likely to attract dirt, as it forms a dry surface. Do not use this type of medication (dry surface) if the wound looks as if it may need to be sutured.

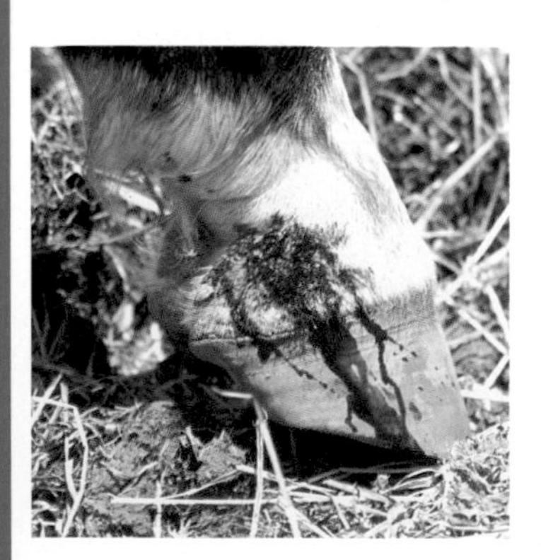

Wounds such as this should be hosed with cool water for 10 minutes before being cleaned.

Call the veterinarian:

- If you have any question about whether the area might require sutures.
- If swelling, heat and pain are not reduced or if they worsen after 24 hours.
- If a pus-like discharge develops or if the edges of a laceration are constantly being pulled apart because of the location of the injury (e.g., over the point of the hock).

Troubleshooting during recovery:
Superficial wounds usually heal uneventfully. Some minor oozing/crusting may be seen and is of no concern. Alert the vet if you see:

- Obvious pus.
- Wounds that were not sutured begin to develop pink tissue (granulation tissue) that extends up higher than skin level.
- Swelling that causes sutures to cut into the skin.
- Wound gaping open between sutures.

DEEP LACERATIONS ■■

Definition:
Deep lacerations penetrate all layers of the skin and are characterized by the edges of the skin gaping apart. There may also be penetration of the injury to the level of the underlying muscle or fascia (covering of muscle), tendons or even bone.

Treatment: *(If bleeding, see Chapter 5, page 48.)*

Laceration through skin only:

- Ideally, suturing needs to be done in the first six hours after the injury occurs. Longer intervals allow bacteria sufficient time to gain entry to the deep layers of tissue.
- Clean the area as described above for superficial wounds. Do not direct forceful streams of water direct-

ly at the wound, as this may cause any dirt to become embedded. Large contaminating objects may be removed safely (e.g., twigs or leaves on the surface), but do not attempt to remove any deep or embedded material — leave this to the veterinarian. When cleaning the wound with gauze, keep to the surface areas but allow the soap to run along the deeper layers.

- Rinse well, directing the water above the wound and allowing it to run over the surface gently.
- Do not apply any spray or wound ointment (unless it's water-based) to the open wound.
- Moisten a sterile gauze dressing with sterile saline solution, if available, and bandage as described above. If you do not have sterile bandaging materials, you may use clean gauze or linen. Do not use cotton fabric or other high-lint materials, as fibers may contaminate the wound. If no lint-free bandaging material is available, it's best to leave the wound uncovered if the veterinarian is expected shortly, or to leave the horse in the wash stall or barn aisle until suitable covering can be obtained.

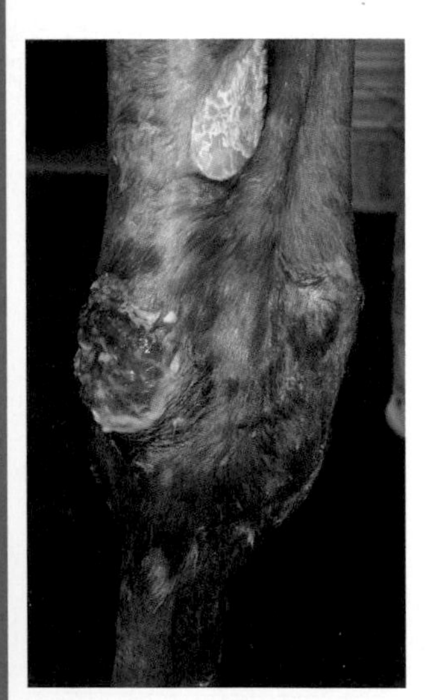

Bandaging around prominent bones in areas with a lot of movement, like the point of the hock, can cause sores.

With deep wounds, dirty wounds, or wounds that are obviously not fresh when first discovered, it is often advisable to give an antibiotic injection immediately. The old standby, for good

Injuries to the coronary band should be evaluated by a vet as soon as possible, for best repair to prevent permanent hoof deformity.

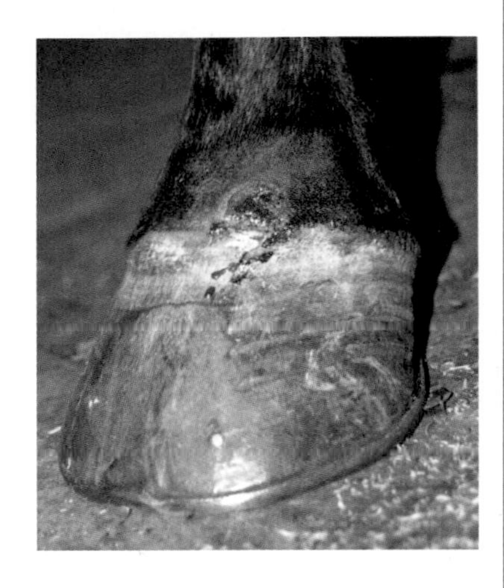

reason, is **procaine penicillin**, but approve with your veterinarian first. These are given intramuscularly. For those uncomfortable with the idea of giving injections, safe oral alternatives include doxycycline or trimethoprim/sulfa which can be added to feed. Before giving any antibiotic, though, get your vet's approval.

- Keep the horse quiet and avoid any unnecessary moving around that could cause bleeding.
- Check on the status of the horse's tetanus immunizations. If he has been vaccinated within the past year, a booster of tetanus toxoid is advisable. If vaccination status is unknown, or the last vaccination was over a year prior to injury, the horse will need both tetanus toxoid and tetanus antitoxin protection. (Antitoxin begins to work immediately.) These may be given at the same time, but not at the same injection site.
- If the horse is trembling, pale, and seems very depressed, blanket him and consult the veterinarian about administering pain medication, such as **phenylbutazone.**

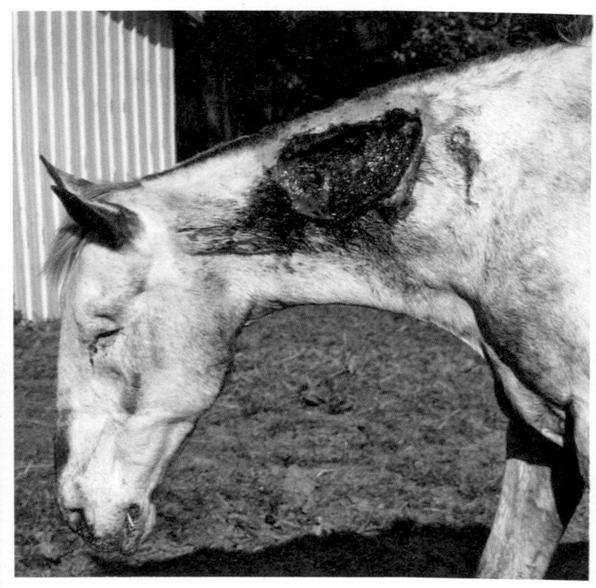

Large gaping wounds like this are extremely painful and will require excellent ongoing care to prevent infection.

Laceration involving skin and muscle:

If the injury penetrates through to the muscular layer, moderate to heavy bleeding often is present and must be controlled first (see Chapter 5, page 42). If it is possible to wash the wound without causing the bleeding to resume at an uncontrolled rate, proceed with cleansing as outlined above. When wounds involve avulsion of muscle — i.e., muscle torn away from its attachments and hanging loose — clean gently as best you can. Then attempt to manipulate the muscle back into the wound cavity, using a moist sponge, and proceed with bandaging. If bandaging is not possible, as with wounds on the chest or high on the hindquarters, stay with the horse to prevent his lying down.

Deep lacerations require immediate veterinary attention to prevent infection.

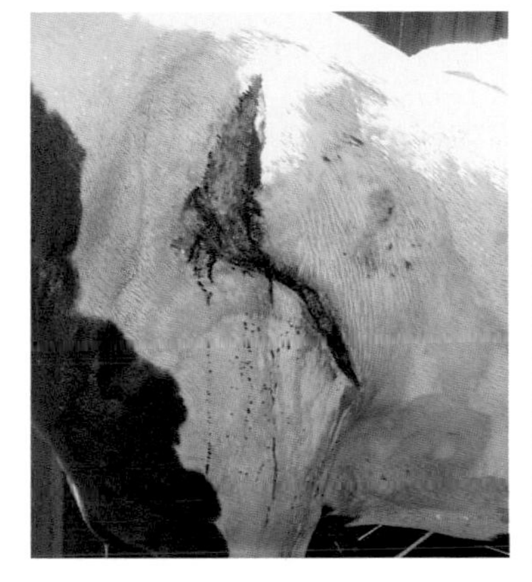

Guidelines for antibiotics, blanketing (not over an open wound), and pain medication are the same as for lacerations through the skin. Again, tetanus status must be ascertained and antitoxin and/or toxoid administered as indicated.

Laceration directly over or within a few inches of a joint or laceration with exposed bone

Any injury near a joint or involving exposed bone is extremely serious. If infection becomes seated in the joint or bone, it can be very difficult, sometimes impossible to treat, and requires extensive and expensive treatment with intravenous antibiotics. Veterinary attention should be obtained within four hours of the injury to maximize the chances of preventing this complication.

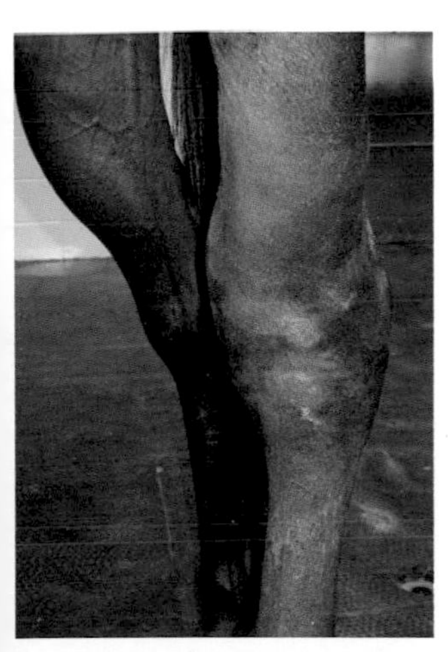

Wounds in the vicinity of joints can progress to joint infections if not properly treated.

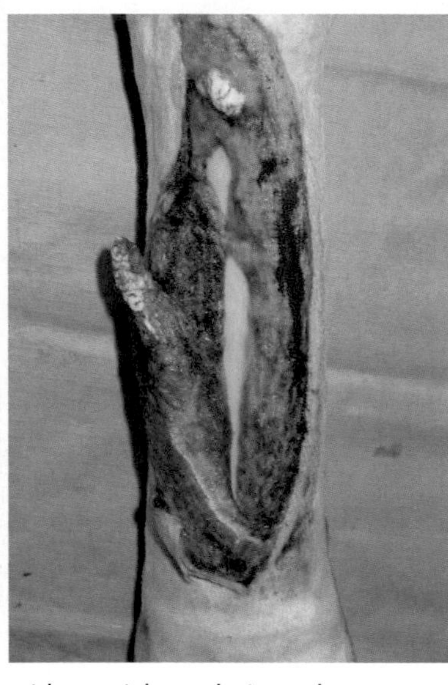

This is a full-thickness cannon bone laceration with exposed bone.

Emergency treatment is the same as for other deep lacerations as outlined above, with special care being taken not to disturb the injured area during cleaning. **Do not move the horse until he's been evaluated by a vet,** as any bone fragments could move and cause more tissue damage or even sever a nerve or vital blood vessel.

Guidelines for bandaging, antibiotics, blanketing and pain medications are the same as for lacerations involving skin and muscles.

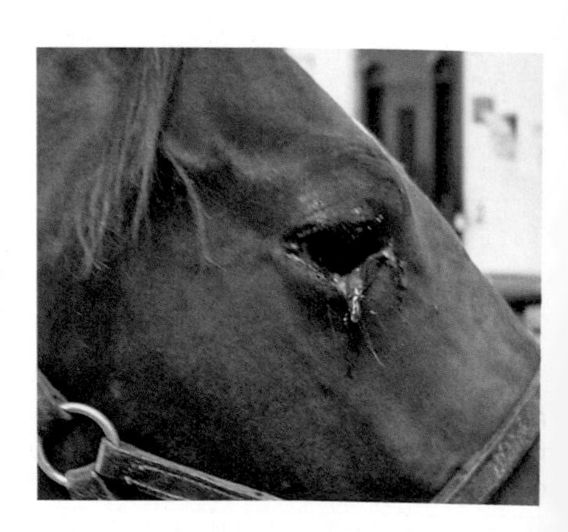

Suturing as soon as possible gives the best odds of returning the eyelid to its original shape and function.

Troubleshooting during recovery:
Wounds involving the deeper tissues have a higher risk of infection. Very extensive wounds may develop areas of skin loss. Alert the vet if you see:

- Skin edges becoming leathery and separating.
- Diffuse swelling or "bubbles" developing under the skin.
- Obvious drainage of pus.
- Swelling that makes the sutures cut into the skin.
- Wound gaping between the sutures.

CONTUSIONS – WITH SKIN INTACT ■ TO ■■

Definition:
A contusion is a blunt injury that does not break the skin but that damages the deep tissues and/or bone. The injured area will show swelling, heat, and tenderness.

Treatment:

- Hose with cold water, 15 to 20 minutes each hour, if possible, or at least three times daily. An alternative is to apply an ice pack under a bandage and leave on for the same amount of time. Severe contusions over the ribs or on the lower legs may have associated fractures. Injury to the abdomen may have caused a defect in the muscles (hernia).

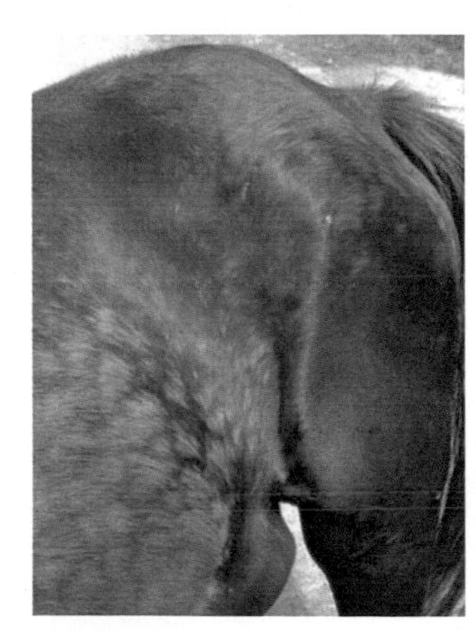

A swelling in this location may be either a hematoma or a hernia.

- Immediate attention should be sought for swellings that are very large or swellings that increase in size (indicating possible bleeding). If there are any signs of colic after an abdominal injury or if the horse shows any signs of shock (depression, trembling, sweating) or internal hemorrhage (white gums), get immediate veterinary attention. Record vital signs initially and at hourly intervals until they are stable (no change for three consecutive readings). If the area can be easily bandaged, apply a bandage between hosing or icing treatments.

Troubleshooting during recovery:
Alert the vet if the amount of swelling increases after the first 24 hours.

PUNCTURE WOUNDS ■■

Definition:
A puncture wound is an invasion of skin and deeper tissues with a relatively small entry point. Nails or other sharp objects can cause puncture wounds.

Treatment:

- If the foot is punctured by a metal object, and the vet is able to make an emergency call within a humane period of time, leave the object in place so X-rays can be taken. They will show exactly how deeply into the foot the nail has penetrated and what structures in the foot have been injured.
- If you can't get the horse seen by a vet within a few hours, or if the object is not metal and the puncture wound is in the foot, grasp the object firmly and pull it straight out. Make a quick sketch of the bottom of the foot with an "X" to mark the spot where the object was located. Save the object to show it to the vet. If the penetrating object fragments when you're trying to remove it, leave it alone for the vet to remove.

If you have to remove the item puncturing the hoof, lest the horse drive it farther into his foot, mark the puncture wound site.

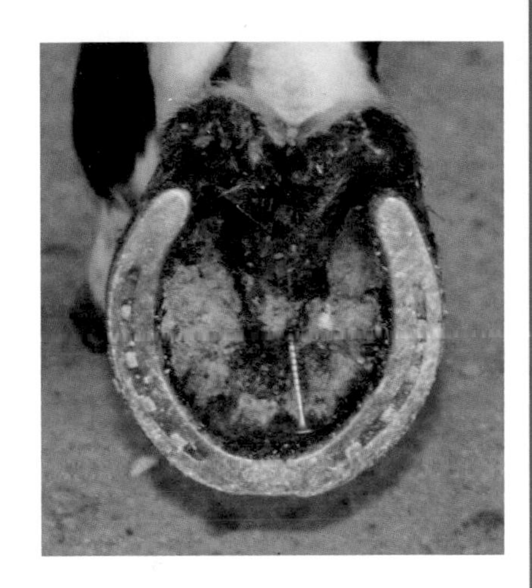

- Heavy bleeding is rare with wounds in the foot (sole or frog area), but some oozing of blood may be seen. The appearance of pus indicates that the wound is old. Clean the foot of debris and manure and soak in hot water with Epsom salts. Administer tetanus toxoid as a booster if the horse has been vaccinated in the past year. If tetanus vaccination status is unknown, ask your vet about the advisability of also giving Tetanus Antitoxin. Do not administer antibiotics. Call the veterinarian to have the wound explored and for any other further treatments recommended.

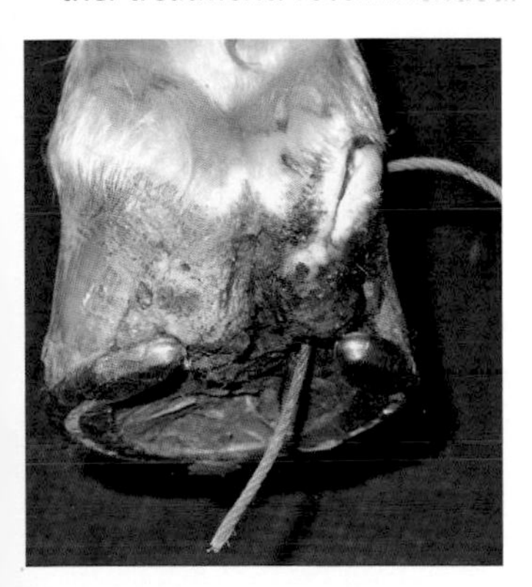

- If the puncture wound is elsewhere on the body and the object is small (such as a nail), grasp it

A good example of how deeply wire can cut into the tissue when a horse gets trapped and struggles.

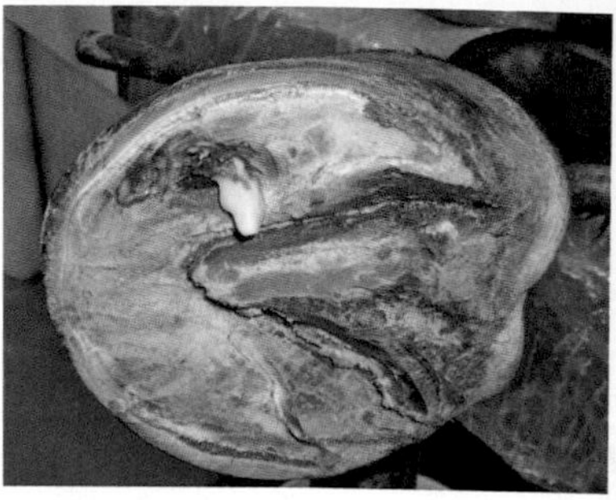

Pus draining from infection at the site of a puncture wound.

firmly and pull it straight out. With other foreign objects, such as glass or wood, it's best to leave extraction to the veterinarian, as hemorrhage may follow removal of a deeply embedded object. Administer tetanus antitoxin/toxoid as described above. Check with the veterinarian before administering antibiotics. Do not flush the depths of a puncture wound prior to veterinary examination — there might be small pieces of debris inside that you could drive in even further.

Troubleshooting during recovery:
Alert the vet if:
- Swelling worsens after the first 24 hours.
- There is obvious drainage of pus.

GUNSHOT WOUNDS ■■■

Definition:
Injuries caused by bullets, pellets, or BBs.

Treatment:
Bleeding may be excessive.
Uncontrolled bleeding, usually arterial bleeding, is called hemorrhage. Attempt to control, as in Chapter 5, page 49. When bleeding is controlled, wash the wound gently as described for lacerations. If bleeding does not stop or if it requires constant pressure for control, don't attempt to clean the wound. Avoid excessive manipulation of the tissues. Administer tetanus protection and antibiotics as advised under lacerations.

Troubleshooting during recovery:
Alert the vet if swelling worsens after first 24 hours or if there is persistent drainage.

SNAKEBITE ■■■

Treatment:

- If the snake has been killed, save it to show the vet. Otherwise, note as many details as you can about the appearance of the snake (but do **not** try to get close for a better look!). If the snake is poisonous, or if you don't know if it is poisonous or not, you need the vet **ASAP**. Even bites from nonpoisonous snakes may swell significantly, so consider any snake bite a reason for a call to the vet.
- Try to keep the horse calm, and if possible, do not move the horse until he's seen by the vet. Poisonous snake bites are rarely fatal in an animal as large as a horse, but systemic complications (e.g., altered blood clotting) can still occur, especially if the bite entered a blood vessel.

Bites on the muzzle/face:

- Bites close to the nostrils can cause enough swelling for them to close off, preventing the horse from breathing. Bites along the undersurface of the head may also swell enough to interfere with breathing.
- With bites to the muzzle, well lubricated (with petroleum jelly or K-Y Jelly), approximately 6-inch-long sections cut from a garden hose can be inserted into one or both nostrils to prevent the swelling from shutting off air. You need to look for the nasal passage opening on the floor of the nostril. Do not insert into the blind pouch that is located along the inner and upper portion of the nostril. This procedure itself is stressful for the horse so observe the horse for a while to see if

swelling is going to progress to this point before attempting it. However, don't wait until swelling has gotten to the point that you can't see what you're doing.

- If the swelling does not involve the muzzle, the nasal tubes won't help. Keep the horse very quiet and still. If swelling progresses to the point the horse is not getting air, see section on tracheostomy.

Bites on the legs:

- While the horse is unlikely to die from a poisonous bite to the legs, there can be very severe tissue damage. Again, a vet needs to see the horse.
- If you are there when the horse is bitten and have bandaging material available, a snug bandage should be placed over the wound using about the same pressure as would be used on a sprain. It should not be tight enough to cut off blood flow, and do not bandage rapidly swelling wounds. A snug, wide band can be applied immediately above the bite to help prevent upward spread of venom, but should not be as tight as a tourniquet. Use about the same amount of pressure as you would in applying a bandage.
- If the bite is not fresh or did not occur while you were there, bandaging won't help. If the bite site is heavily contaminated with dirt or manure, you can gently wash it with soap and water. Cold can help control swelling, but opinions vary on the advisability of using ice because there may be so much tissue damage that the area will be more sensitive to cold. The best approach is to run cold water over the leg until the vet gets there. If the vet instructs you to do so, give tetatnus toxoid or antitoxin.
- Do **not** cut the wound, squeeze the wound, suck on the wound or use suction cups.

Troubleshooting during recovery:
The first 4 to 12 hours are most critical in terms of swelling and systemic complications.

- The horse should be observed constantly for signs of breathing difficulties, worsening swelling, red or brown urine (from red cell destruction or muscle breakdown). If these are seen, call the vet back immediately.
- Horses with bites to the head/face may not be able to drink. If the horse tries to drink but you can't see him swallow, call the vet. Arrangements will have to be made for intravenous fluids or fluids by stomach tube.

After the first 4 to 12 hours, things to look for are the same as for any puncture wound.

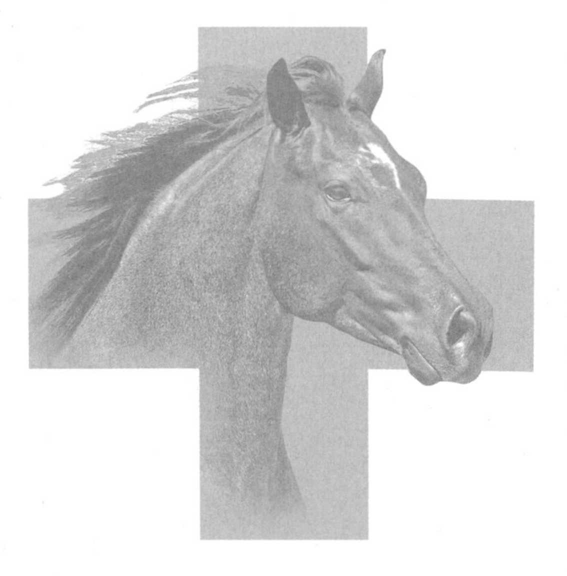

05

BLEEDING

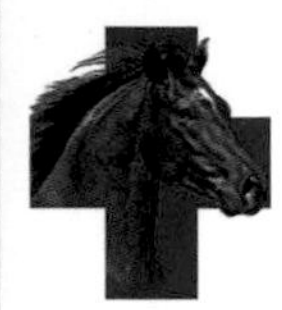

FIRST AID KIT

- Gauze pads
- Quilted leg wraps
- Elasticized leg wraps
- Electrolytes
- Belt or tourniquet
- Tranquilizer ℞
- Blanket
- Tetanus toxoid ℞
- Tetanus antitoxin ℞
- Twitch
- Injectable or oral antibiotics ℞

℞: PRESCRIPTION DRUG — MUST BE OBTAINED FROM VETERINARIAN OR PRESCRIBED BY A VET — SHOULD NEVER BE ADMINISTERED WITHOUT PRIOR APPROVAL BY A VETERINARIAN.

QUICK CHAPTER REFERENCE LIST

LEGEND: ■■■ — NEEDS EMERGENCY ATTENTION; ■■ — SHOULD BE EXAMINED BY A VET;
■ — MAY NEED VETERINARY ADVICE/ATTENTION

BLEEDING

A horse's body holds in the neighborhood of 8 to 9 gallons of blood. The horse will go into shock if he loses about 25 percent of that (2 to 2.5 gallons). Quantifying how much blood is being lost is always difficult, but it's important to at least try so you can let the vet know what's going on. Note such things as:

- Size of any pools/puddles of blood.
- If the area below the wound is saturated with blood.
- If blood is actively spurting from the wound under pressure or is more of a steady ooze/drain.
- How long it takes a bandage to get saturated with blood.

> Caution: **Always contact the vet for any bleeding that does not stop spontaneously within 10 minutes,** or bleeding that is not from an obvious cause, such as a wound.

FROM WOUNDS

Oozing ■

Oozing is a slow leak or trickle of blood, caused by damage to superficial vessels.

Treatment:

- Apply clean gauze or lint-free material to the surface of the wound.
- Apply pressure for three to five minutes.
- Proceed with treatment as detailed in Chapter 4, page 29 for the type of injury and area injured.

When wounds do not involve large veins or arteries, bleeding from cut skin edges and deeper tissues eventually stops after the vessels contract and clots form.

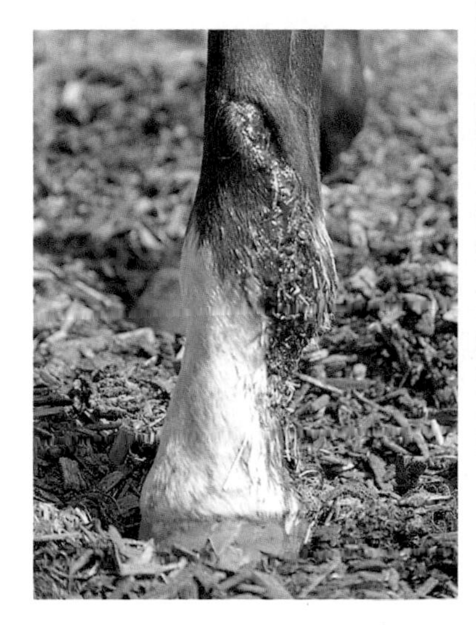

Venous bleeding ■■

Bleeding from veins will vary from minimal to profuse, depending on the size of the blood vessel(s) involved and the area injured. Venous bleeding will stop easily when sufficient pressure is applied. The red color of venous blood is not as bright as the red color of arterial blood.

Treatment:

- Apply clean gauze or lint-free bandage material to the surface of the wound.
- Hold bandage in place by hand or wrap for a minimum of five minutes. Press lightly but firmly, with the same amount of pressure it takes to leave a white spot on the back of your hand. If bleeding resumes when pressure is removed, reapply for another five minutes. If bandages soak through quickly, suspect arterial bleeding.

Arterial bleeding ■■■

Arterial bleeding is profuse, brisk, and bright red. If the artery is located close to the surface, the characteristic pulsations may be seen (spurts). With deep arterial bleeding, pulsations may not be obvious, but the wound cavity will fill with blood quickly. With deep arterial bleeding, tissues surrounding the wound may also swell rapidly.

Treatment:

- Apply clean gauze or lint-free bandage material to the surface of the wound. Hold the bandage in place by hand, or wrap it.
- If possible, apply a tourniquet with just enough pressure to stop the bleeding. Release the tourniquet briefly (for approximately 30 to 60 seconds) every 5 minutes.
- If the bleeding stops, proceed with wound care. If bleeding does not stop, or it resumes heavily again when you try to clean the wound, continue pressure until vet arrives.

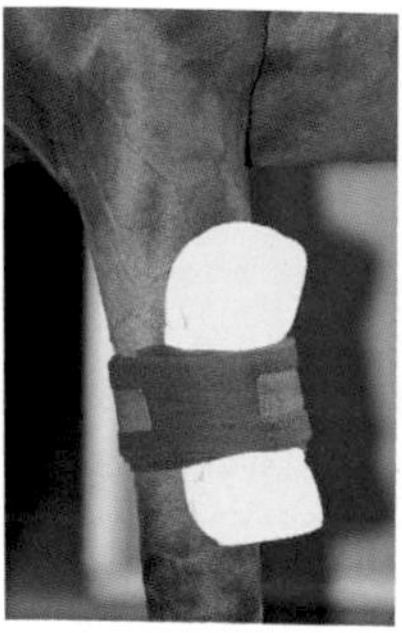

Pressure wrap.

Trouble shooting during recovery:
Wounds that bled heavily sometimes start bleeding again within the 24 hours following repair. If the vet advised keeping the area wrapped, do not change the wrap for the first 24 hours unless you see blood has soaked through to the outer bandage. If the wound is not wrapped, watch it and call the vet if marked swelling develops under the skin or if the wound itself starts to leak blood.

FROM NOSE

After exercise ■■

Bleeding from the nose may be coming from the upper respiratory tract or from the lungs. The cause may be either the stress of exercise or an underlying disease or infection.

Treatment:

- Record vital signs every five minutes until there's no change for three consecutive readings.
- If the horse is overheated, sponge him with tepid water and apply a light sheet. Keep the horse quiet.
- If the bleeding does not slow significantly in five minutes or if it is extremely profuse, try elevating the head slightly (you can do this by putting the horse on crossties). But if the horse has trouble breathing or makes choking noises, release the head immediately.

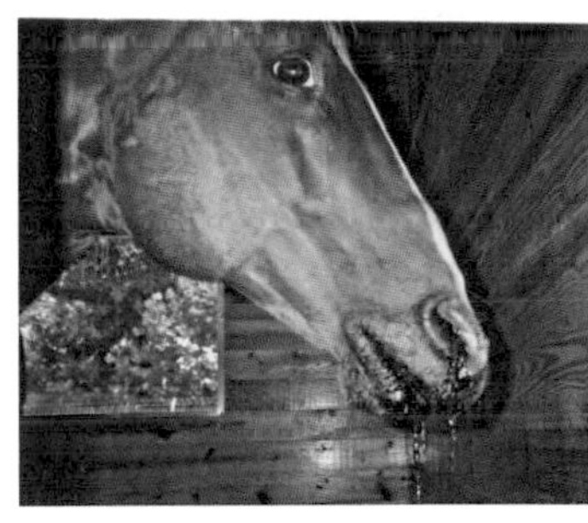

Do not attempt to pack the horse's nose if there is a bloody discharge.

- Do not tranquilize the horse without obtaining permission from the veterinarian first. Do not attempt to pack the nose.

After injury to the head ■■■

Fracture is possible. Since the head has a rich supply of blood vessels, this type of bleeding could be life-threatening.

Treatment:

- Record vital signs every five minutes.
- If horse is trembling and shaky, blanket him appropriately according to the weather.
- Do **not** raise his head or attempt to pack the nose. You may administer pain medication after getting veterinary approval.
- Do not tranquilize the horse unless recommended by a veterinarian.
- Place the horse in a quiet stall and avoid undue handling.

Reason unknown ■■■

May be caused by an unwitnessed injury, an infection, or a disorder of blood clotting.

Treatment:

- Record vital signs every five minutes or until the bleeding stops.
- Note any unusual behavior or unusual color to the mucous membranes.
- Do not give any medications.
- Blanket the horse according to the weather. Place him in a quiet stall and avoid undue handling.

FROM EARS

After injury to head ■■■

Cause: Probably skull fracture.

Treatment:

See Chapter 15, page 153. There's nothing you can do about bleeding from the ear. Do not try to pack the ear. Keep the horse quiet. Call the vet immediately.

Reason unknown ■■

If the reason for bleeding from the ear(s) is unknown, strongly suspect trauma. There may be a deep injury to the ear. Blanket the horse as necessary according to the weather. Place him in a quiet stall and avoid undue handling. Record vital signs when the injury is first detected, but then do not disturb him. Watch for any unusual behavior such as tilting the head, pressing the head against the wall or difficulty with balance. Call the vet.

From wound to ear ■

Treatment:

Treat as for any other laceration. If the tissue is torn through, avoid excessive pulling. The horse will probably require tranquilization or twitching. If resistance is violent, await arrival of the veterinarian.

FROM MOUTH ■■■

Cause: Probable injury to gums or tongue. Bleeding from tongue may be very profuse. Do not panic at the amount of blood.

Treatment:

- Thoroughly rinse mouth with cold water until no grain or hay material is flushed out.
- Remove hay and grain from stall, but allow access to water (horse may soak or rinse mouth himself).
- Record vital signs every 10 minutes until stable.
- Call the vet.

> **Trouble shooting during recovery:**
> Follow your vet's instructions regarding what to feed (usually soft meals). If you're feeding hay, soak it thoroughly first. If heavy bleeding occurs again, remove all feed and call the vet.

With bleeding from nose ■■■

Heavy bleeding from throat area or deeper is the probable cause.

Treatment:

- Record vital signs every five minutes.
- Blanket him according to the weather, and avoid undue disturbance.
- Call the vet if the bleeding doesn't stop in 10 minutes.

FROM OTHER BODY ORIFICES

From anus or vagina following breeding ■■■

Cause: Probable rupture of vagina or rectum

Treatment:

- Record vital signs every five minutes.
- Blanket as necessary if the horse shows signs of shock.
- According to vet's instructions, administer tetanus toxoid if the horse has been vaccinated within the past year; administer both tetanus toxoid and antitoxin if the vaccination status is unknown or if vaccination occurred over a year ago.
- Administer antibiotics after veterinary approval. Keep the horse quiet.

From vagina only ■■ to ■■■

Suspect sadism, varicose veins or accidental injury. Treat as above. (For bloody urine, see Chapter 19, page 185.)

From anus only ■■■

Cause: Probable sadism or freak injury. Tumor is a distant possibility. Blood may also be seen with severe intestinal infections when there will be associated diarrhea.

Treatment:

- If diarrhea is not present, treat as for bleeding following breeding (see above). If diarrhea is present as well, tell the veterinarian, and treat as for diarrhea.

From penis ■■ to ■■■

See chapters on Reproductive Organs (Chapter 20, page 189) and Disorders of Urine/Urination (Chapter 19, page 183).

06

BURNS

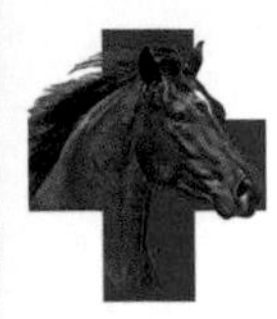

FIRST AID KIT

- Mild soap
- Silver sulfadiazine cream
- Sterile gauze pads
- Antibacterial ointment
- Antibiotic injection ℞ (if ordered by veterinarian based on culture results)
- Cold pack
- A & D ointment
- Zinc oxide
- Aloe
- Lavender oil
- Skin Rejuvenator/ Veterinus Derma-Gel

℞: PRESCRIPTION DRUG — MUST BE OBTAINED FROM VETERINARIAN OR PRESCRIBED BY A VET — SHOULD NEVER BE ADMINISTERED WITHOUT PRIOR APPROVAL BY A VETERINARIAN.

QUICK CHAPTER REFERENCE LIST

LEGEND: ■■■ — NEEDS EMERGENCY ATTENTION; ■■ — SHOULD BE EXAMINED BY A VET; ■ — MAY NEED VETERINARY ADVICE/ATTENTION

BURNS

Burns may be caused by heat, electricity, or chemicals.

Chemical burns are relatively rare in horses, the most common being accidental contact of the skin with caustic chemicals, like strong copper sulfate solutions used to control thrush or fungal hoof infections. Improper dilution (too concentrated) of fly spray concentrates can also cause chemical burns, as can inappropriate or overly aggressive use of leg paints that contain iodine or mercury. Even herbal essential oils can cause chemical burns if applied as the pure oil. Severe skin reactions to topicals are chemical burns.

SUPERFICIAL BURNS ■

Definition:
A superficial burn is characterized by reddening and swelling of the skin, but the skin is not open. Animals rarely show blister formation.

Treatment:

- Clip hair for a generous distance around the burn to better define the extent of the damage.
- If the burn is caused by chemicals, spray the area with a rapidly running stream of cold water for at least 15 minutes. Then gently clean with mild soap and water.
- Do the same for electrical or flame burns, except don't use soap. For other superficial burns, hose the area with cold water for 15 minutes every hour for the first 24 hours, or use a cold pack for same amount of time.
- Chemical burns should also be treated with cold therapy for 15 minutes out of every hour for the first 24

hours. This may seem like a great deal of work, but burns can cause extensive problems that might not show up for several days. The best way to control the local inflammation and tissue damage that occurs with burns is with cold. It also provides significant pain relief. If the skin eventually cracks/opens or dies and is lost, treat as below.

Troubleshooting during recovery:
Superficial burns may not show the full extent of damage for 72 hours. Watch carefully for the development of leathery skin. If this occurs, leave it in place as a natural bandage. Skin will grow in underneath the damaged layer. Alert the vet if any drainage develops

DEEP BURNS ■■■

Definition:
A burn that has a break in the skin surface as soon as the injury occurs, or a burn that appears to be intact initially, but starts oozing or sloughing off a few days later.

Treatment:

- Direct a generous stream of rapidly running, cool water at the burn for 10 to 15 minutes.
- Gently, but thoroughly, clean the area with mild soap (Ivory, glycerin, green soap) and warm water to remove all dead tissue. (Note: The warm water is only

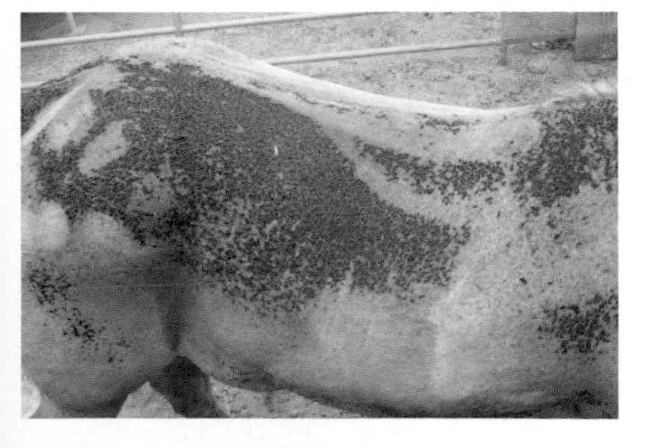

This significant burn could easily be mistaken for a dirty coat.

to remove soap residue.) However, do not forcefully pull on any areas where the skin is still attached.

- Rinse thoroughly with cool water. Allow the burn to dry. Then apply an antibacterial cream such as silver sulfadiazine, (which is the antibacterial treatment of choice). If this isn't available, you may use a light coating of zinc oxide, A & D cream or ointment, or other antibacterial wound cream in the interim. Pure aloe gel, with a few drops of lavender oil as a gentle anesthetic, also makes an excellent burn treatment, as does Veterinus derma-gel, an herbal-based ointment that encourages healing and has pain-relieving properties.

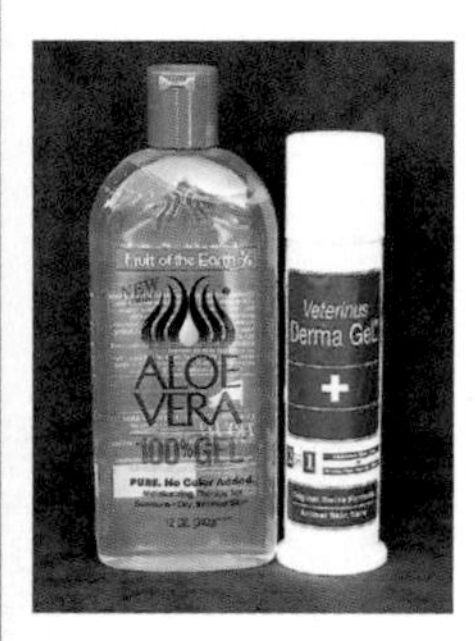

- A light bandage of sterile gauze or Telfa may be used. Do not bandage heavily. Clean and dress the area once a day, more often if the burn becomes dirty, drains heavily or if an unbandaged wound dries out.

Troubleshooting during recovery:
Alert the vet if you don't see reduction in the size of the open area on a daily basis or if the above measures are not successful in stopping drainage or eliminating pus.

Burn Complications:

- **Scarring:** Deep burns may scar badly, particularly if they cover a large area. Skin grafting may be required after the area heals.
- **Infection:** When burns break the skin, infection is always a risk. The best prevention is faithful treatment, as above. Monitor the horse's rectal temperature at least twice daily or any time the animal appears depressed until the burn heals. Consult a veterinarian before starting any oral or injectable antibiotics.

- **Shock:** Burns covering a large surface area may result in the loss of fluids through oozing. This fluid loss may be sufficient to cause shock. Call the vet immediately if you sense the horse is going into shock. Signs of shock include:
  — weakness
  — trembling
  — depression
  — cold ears and extremities
  — a rapid, but weak pulse
  — pale mucous membranes with prolonged capillary refill time.

  Monitor for shock by looking for the above signs carefully during the first three days after an extensive burn injury. Record vital signs every hour for the first 24 hours, and four times daily after that or any time the animal seems worse. The horse should continue to drink within his normal range (12 to 20 gallons a day). He may urinate less when in shock. Veterinary coverage is advisable from the start when burns are extensive.

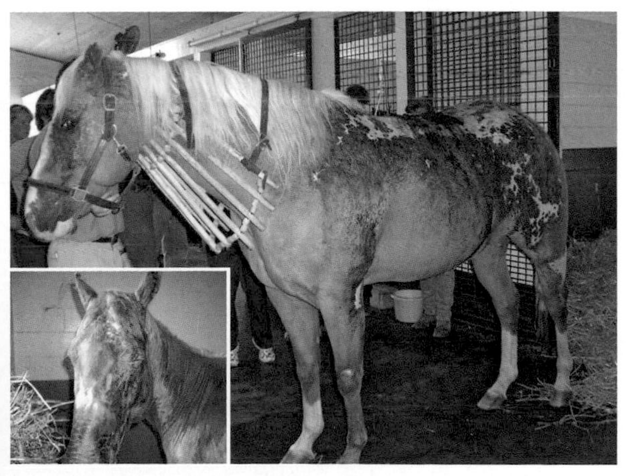

This horse was severly burned but with good veterinary care, he's mending well. Photos taken one year apart.

- **Kidney damage:** Shock may have associated kidney shutdown, so be especially observant of water consumption and urination in animals with extensive burns. Keep track of how many buckets of water are consumed a day, and how wet the stall is compared to normal. Alert the vet immediately if decreased urinary output is suspected. Liver damage may accompany kidney failure.
- **Lung damage:** Respiratory difficulty may be a late complication of animals trapped in fires or suffering from electrical burns. Observe the horse for increased respiratory rate, noisy breathing, difficult/labored breathing and froth at the nose or mouth. Call the vet immediately if lung damage is suspected.

07

DISORDERS OF EATING/COLIC

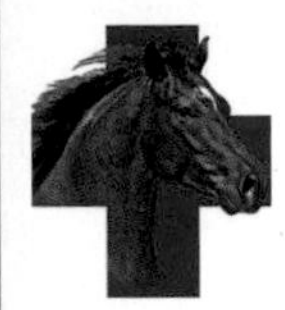

FIRST AID KIT

- Acepromazine ℞
- Table salt
- Peroxide
- Flunixin meglumine (Banamine) ℞
- Xylazine (Rompun) ℞
- Potassium chloride (salt substitute)
- Baking soda or Alka-Seltzer
- Disinfectant
- Mineral oil

℞: PRESCRIPTION DRUG — MUST BE OBTAINED FROM VETERINARIAN OR PRESCRIBED BY A VET — SHOULD NEVER BE ADMINISTERED WITHOUT PRIOR APPROVAL BY A VETERINARIAN.

QUICK CHAPTER REFERENCE LIST

LEGEND: ■■■ — NEEDS EMERGENCY ATTENTION; ■■ — SHOULD BE EXAMINED BY A VET; ■ — MAY NEED VETERINARY ADVICE/ATTENTION

DISORDERS OF EATING/COLIC

SALIVATION/DROOLING ■ to ■■■

Causes (partial list):

- Choke — blockage of esophagus by food.
- Paralysis of throat, as with botulism, lead poisoning or rabies.
- Tetanus.
- Irritation of mouth from ingestion of plant or insect.
- Injury or tumor of mouth or throat.

Diagnosis:

- **Choke** is most common in older animals during cold weather when water intake may be limited, and in horses fed coarse hays, pelleted feeds and/or corn on the cob. Mashes and soaked feeds may cause choke if they are eaten rapidly. Repeated attempts to swallow may be noted, and the horse may seem to be gagging. Careful palpation along the neck in the groove where the jugular vein lies will often reveal a hard lump, which is the blockage. Blockage may also occur in the lower parts of the esophagus, within the chest.
- As in all cases when **rabies** is a possibility, rabies should be carefully considered before approaching the horse. **If the horse is showing any signs of nervous system disturbance, such as hyperexcitability, sensitivity to sound, or seizures, do not attempt an examination.**
- With **botulism**, there will also be signs of generalized muscle weakness and staggering. Movement of the tail by hand will often show there is little tone or resistance

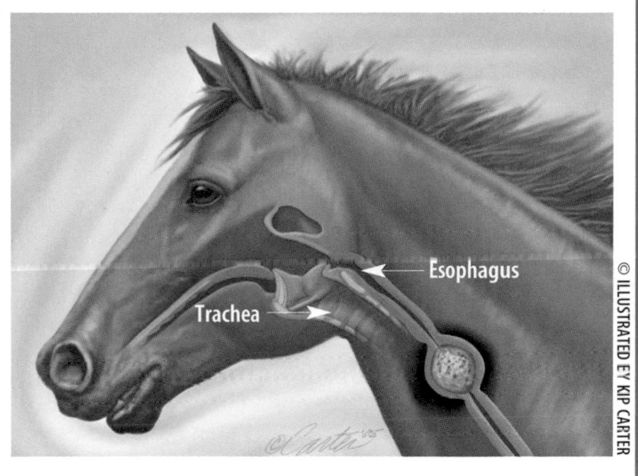

© ILLUSTRATED BY KIP CARTER

Choke in horses involves food getting stuck/impacted in the esophagus, the tube leading to the stomach. Symptoms are saliva dripping from the mouth because the horse can't swallow it, and sometimes retching or gagging-type movements. Unlike choking in people, the trachea, tube leading to the lungs, is not blocked so the horse can still breathe.

to manipulation. Anal tone is decreased. With **lead poisoning**, there is also paralysis of the muscles of the larynx, leading to a dramatic "roaring" noise on respiration with exercise or excitement. Weakness, staggering and swollen joints may be present.

- **Tetanus** is characterized by the horse's inability to open his mouth and a very stiff, "sawhorse" stance with rigidity of the tail.
- **Irritation, injury or tumor** of the mouth or throat may be visible on inspection with a flashlight. Pull the horse's tongue to one side to make him keep his mouth open, while you examine his mouth.

Treatment:

- **Choke**:
  — Place the horse in a quiet stall without bedding.

— Allow access to water but remove any feed or grain. Obstructions will sometimes pass on their own.
— Mild tranquilization with Acepromazine is helpful (20 to 30 mg. intramuscularly for a 1,000-pound horse), but get approval from your vet first. When the horse is tranquilized, remove the water from the stall.

Get veterinary attention:

- If the obstruction is not relieved within 30 minutes.
- If there is a foul odor to the breath.
- If you are unsure how long the esophagus has been obstructed.

Delay in relieving the obstruction can result in serious damage to the esophagus and permanent problems. (CAUTION: it is possible for the obstructing lump to disappear from the neck only to become lodged again at the point the esophagus enters the chest. You will not be able to feel it, but the horse will still be unable to move materials into his stomach. Persistence of salivation and refusal to eat or drink will indicate this has happened.)

Troubleshooting during recovery:

- Horses that bolt their food without chewing it well are at higher risk of choke because insufficient chewing decreases the amount of saliva swallowed with the food. Avoid pelleted feed and/or put a few rounded rocks in the feed tub to force the horse to pick around them and get smaller mouthfuls.
- Older horses that choke may have problems with chewing due to poor teeth and/or neurological problems with swallowing. Consult with your vet about the advisability of going to a soaked complete feed.

- **Suspected botulism, lead poisoning or tetanus**:
  If salivation is accompanied by general muscle weakness, decreased anal tone, "roaring," staggering, swollen joints, an inability to open the mouth or a stiff stance, get immediate veterinary attention. Avoid moving or stimulating the horse in any way.

- **Mechanical or insect irritation**:
  If the mouth looks very reddened or an obvious area(s) of injury or ulceration can be found, flush the mouth with generous amounts of cold water (using a hose) to loosen any debris or food in the mouth and to provide some pain relief. Allow access to water, but no hay or grain for 4 to 8 hours. Rinse the mouth every two hours with warm salt water (about 2 tablespoons/quart) or diluted peroxide solution (about a 10-percent solution). The mucosa in this area heals quickly. Offer a mash after 8 to 12 hours.

  Troubleshooting during recovery:
  If the horse is not drinking, get veterinary attention immediately. If the horse refuses to eat for longer than 8 to 12 hours, get veterinary attention.

- **Wound or tumor of mouth or throat**:
  Extensive injuries should receive immediate veterinary attention to prevent the development of complications. Do not attempt to flush out any wounds when the horse is not swallowing well, as he could inhale the fluid. If breathing problems develop, see Chapter 12, page 123. Remove all food and water and keep the horse quiet.

  Troubleshooting during recovery:
  Call the vet if the horse is drinking less than 5 gallons/day, or is not eating the recommended diet well.

POOR APPETITE ■ to ■■■

Causes:

Poor appetite may be observed any time the horse is under physical (pain, illness) or emotional stress, if the hay or grain you are feeding is not wholesome, and as a symptom of a digestive tract problem. Horses with gastric (stomach) ulcers will often eat less grain and prefer hay or grass. Foals with stomach ulcers may stop eating entirely.

Treatment:

Find the cause of the poor appetite.

- Carefully examine the grain and hay for off smells, colors or textures.
- Take the horse's temperature, pulse, and respiratory rate.
- Examine the legs and feet for any heat or swelling, and watch the horse move.
- Be alert for development of more specific signs of an intestinal problem (see below).

Troubleshooting during recovery:

If you cannot determine the cause, call the vet. The horse should go back on good feed/hay immediately if the cause was spoiled hay or poor quality diet. For what to expect after treatment of a digestive problem, see below.

REFUSAL TO EAT/DRINK ■■

Refusal to eat or drink is a non-specific sign that something is seriously wrong. It may be caused by an inability to eat or drink (see above), or by abdominal pain (see colic, below). However, anything that causes severe pain or makes the horse very ill can result in refusal to eat or drink. You should record the vital signs (temperature,

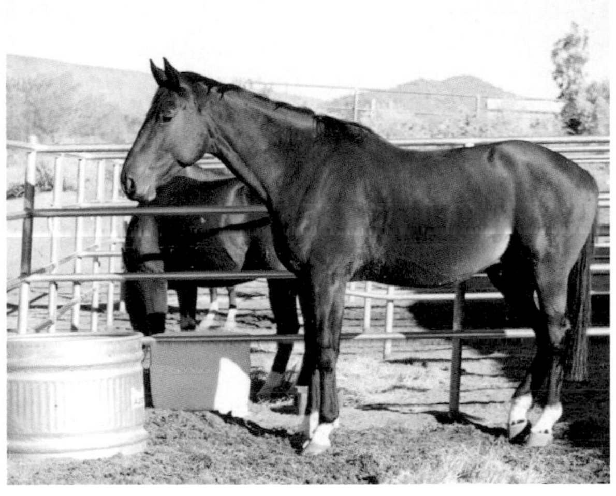

Even if the horse stops eating, he may play with his water, giving you the impression that he's drinking. Refusal of feed and water is a serious sign.

pulse, respiration) as a first step. Think of any recent stresses that could have caused a problem (long shipping, heavy exercise, etc.) and observe for other symptoms that may indicate where the problem lies. Call the vet for examination and specific treatment.

Troubleshooting during recovery:
Horses treated for gastric ulcers usually show a much better appetite within 2 to 3 days. Horses recovering from colic vary in their recovery times depending on the problem. Ask your vet when to expect your horse to recover his appetite. Stressed horses should be back on feed within 3 days. Horses not eating because of pain will resume eating when their pain is adequately controlled.

FOOD/WATER COMING OUT THE NOSE ■ to ■■

Causes:

In foals, this may be a sign of cleft palate. In adult horses, food may occasionally come out the nose if the horse becomes excited and does not swallow properly when eating. Otherwise, problems with the soft palate, choke or paralysis somewhere in the throat can cause this problem. Temporary difficulties may develop during severe upper-respiratory infections.

Treatment:

- Foals should be examined and treated for cleft palate as soon as possible. The presence of food along the nasal passages can result in irritation and severe infections, including pneumonia.
- With adults, if the horse regularly has food appearing at his nostrils when eating, bring this to your vet's attention. It's likely not an emergency.
- With respiratory infections, the problem may resolve itself as the throat returns to normal.

Troubleshooting during recovery:

If large amounts of food or water coming from the nose is a continuing problem, and particularly if any abnormal discharge appears, a veterinarian should examine the area with an endoscope to locate the problem and suggest treatment.

COUGHING/CHOKING WHEN EATING ■ to ■■

Causes:

Coughing or choking during eating may be caused by allergies to the grain or hay, irritation of the throat by infection, a structural abnormality or paralysis of the throat area.

Treatment:

- If the problem develops suddenly after switching to a new (possibly dusty or moldy) grain or hay or if the coughing occurs only when the barn is closed up tightly, suspect an allergy. Go back to feed you know is well tolerated or try wetting down the hay or grain slightly before feeding.
- Problems that develop during a known respiratory infection will usually be self-limiting. You can make things easier by substituting a mash for dry grains during this time and avoiding coarse hays, even if there is not a classical "cold" syndrome going on.
- Two- to three-year-old horses may have deep seated infections in the lymphatic tissues of their throats that will often cause this problem. These horses, as well as any horses without any obvious identifiable cause for the problem, should be examined with an endoscope.

Troubleshooting during recovery:
If the above measures don't correct the problem, call your vet.

COLIC ■■ to ■■■

Definition:
Colic is a term used to describe abdominal pain of any origin.

Symptoms:
The horse with colic will show different signs, depending on the severity and nature of the problem. In mild cases:

- The horse is depressed.
- The head is lowered.
- Breathing is somewhat rapid.
- Pulse is normal or slightly elevated.
- The horse may look back at his flanks or bite at his flanks.
- A male may drop his penis.
- Appetite is poor or absent, although the horse may drink or play with the water.

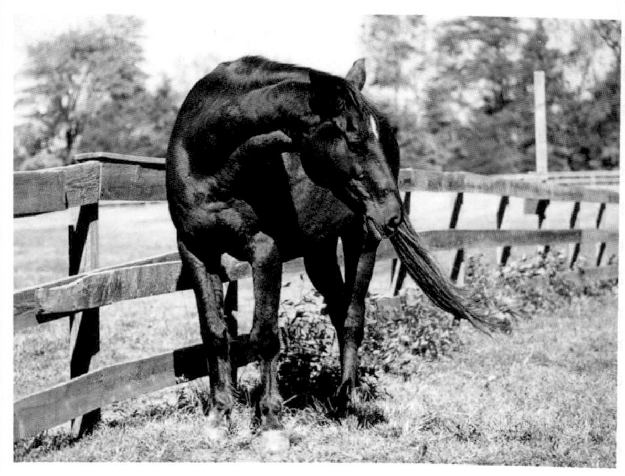

Early signs of colic may be depression, restlessness or the horse may look back at or kick at his belly.

- Manure may be absent or abnormal (diarrhea, hard balls with mucus, etc.).

As the severity of the problem increases, so does the pain. Horses then begin to show:

- Sweating
- Pawing
- Pacing
- Blowing respirations
- Markedly elevated pulse
- Discolored mucus membranes (bright red or bluish)
- Desire to lie down and roll or thrash.

Causes:

Mild cases of colic may be caused by heavy parasite burdens, either in the intestine or stomach or immature forms in the arteries; by old damage from heavy parasite burdens; or by changes in routine, exercise, or feed that cause altered eating patterns. Mild colic may stem from impaction, indigestion, gastric ulcers, diarrhea, or spasmodic colic — a condition where a portion of intestine is in spasm, preventing food and gas from traveling on and resulting in distension of the intestine and pain.

Severe cases of colic are usually related to the loss of blood supply to a section of intestine, severe infection/inflammation of the intestine, complete blockage of fecal material and gas from ingestion of foreign material such as rubber fencing, etc., or to twisting or malposition of a section of intestine that also causes a complete blockage. In these cases, the horse's system also becomes "toxic" as bacterial products are absorbed across the bowel wall. The mucous membranes become bright red or bluish, the ear and legs are often cold, and founder (laminitis) may set in as a complication (see Chapter 9, page 100.)

Treatment:

With all colic cases, getting organized is the first step. This will give the vet valuable information, should he/she be needed, and will also provide you a clear idea of the horse's progress. Don't rely on your memory or vague impressions to make decisions in a colic case. Keep track of the horse's symptoms and the times you observe them. (The form on page 325 may be helpful.)

- Mild cases of colic often respond to walking or turning the horse out. Walking is advised at first so that you can monitor the horse.
- Once he has passed gas and manure and seems interested in eating, it's safe to turn the horse out.
- Avoid grain for the next 24 hours. Keep hay, salt and water available.
- Observe the horse frequently over the next 24 hours for signs of recurrence, and be aware that colic is something an individual horse may be prone to develop.
- Mild cases that don't respond to walking alone will need medication. Call your vet for advice and dosages before giving any medications to a horse with colic.

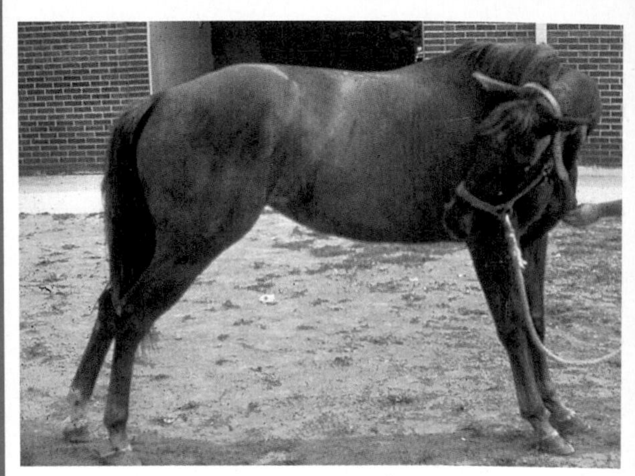

Horses with colic or laminitis may assume the stretched out, "sawhorse" stance. This horse has colic and is looking back at this flanks.

Any horse that needs medication should also probably be examined by the vet.

- Banamine is highly recommended for treatment of colic, and may be all that is needed in mild cases. The dose is 0.5 mg./lb. once or twice daily.
- Acepromazine, 25 to 30 mg. (for a 1,000-pound horse), given intramuscularly can help relieve intestinal spasms. Do not give acepromazine until the veterinarian has been informed of the horse's vital signs and symptoms (which could indicate impending or present shock) and has approved the use of this drug.

As already mentioned, severe pain is the most reliable indicator available to an owner that the horse may have a serious condition. Although horses vary in their ability to withstand pain, any horse showing violent pawing, rolling, and thrashing needs immediate veterinary attention. In the interim, proceed in the same manner as listed for the treatment of mild colic. However, you should give a tranquilizer as well if the horse is very agitated and difficult to handle. As above, acepromazine may help relieve intestinal spasms and is also an effective tranquilizer. Rompun at 1 mg./lb. intramuscularly is also a good choice. The effect will last one to two hours. Don't use tranquilizers without prior veterinary approval.

Leave the horse alone after injection (unless he's rolling and thrashing violently, in which case you want to try to keep him standing.) After the horse has calmed down, proceed as outlined above. If the horse is in a great deal of distress, it may be best to let him stand quietly rather than trying to force him to walk, which could make him attempt to throw himself to the ground.

As a final note on severe colic, the sudden and unexplained appearance of an apparent improvement with reduced pain can be a severe sign. This often signals that a segment of intestine has ruptured. The apparent relief is due to reduced pressure along the gut. Contact your veterinarian for advice immediately.

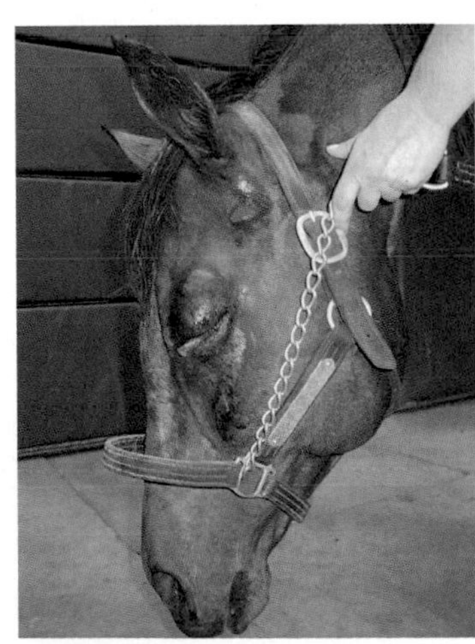

Horses in severe pain, panicking in situations where they are trapped, or horses with encephalitis can do severe damage to their own heads when they thrash around.

Troubleshooting during recovery:

With mild colic cases, it's time to get a visit from the veterinarian if:

- The horse fails to respond to walking or medications recommended by the vet.
- The condition worsens, as indicated by:
  - — Increasing pulse and respiration.
  - — Worsening pain and agitation.
  - — Failure to pass manure for 12 hours or longer. Note whether the horse is passing gas or not. Small amounts of liquid may pass a large impaction; don't be fooled by this.
  - — Passage of abnormal manure, or diarrhea that doesn't return to normal in one or two bowel movements.
  - — Development of signs of laminitis.

DIARRHEA ■■

Definition:

An increase in the frequency of manure passage or in the amount of manure. In the horse, diarrhea generally means a change in manure from well-formed balls to soft or liquid feces.

Causes:

There are many causes of diarrhea, including

- Stress
- Parasites
- Alteration in the normal populations of bacteria and other microorganisms in the gut due to antibiotics
- Change in hay or grain, excessive grass intake
- May be related to infections of the intestines (such as salmonella).

Complications:

Dehydration. Laminitis, commonly known as founder, is possible (see chapter 9, page 100).

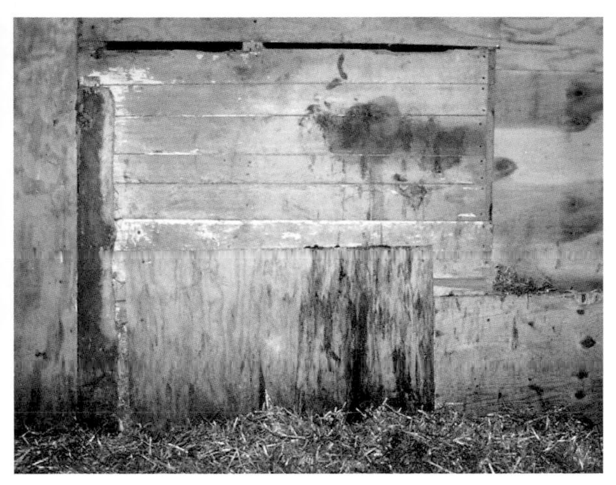

Observe the stall and manure for signs of diarrhea.

Treatment:

Treat symptoms of diarrhea as described above for mild colic.

- Avoid alfalfa.
- Keep fresh water in constant supply.
- Offer a second bucket containing an electrolyte mixture, either a commercially available pre-mixed powder or one you make up containing:

  2 oz. table salt

  1 oz. potassium chloride (salt substitute)

  1 oz. baking soda (or 10 plain Alka-Seltzer tablets)

  Add the above to five gallons of water.
- Since there is always the possibility of salmonella infection, which is a hazard to both humans and other animals, a horse with diarrhea should be kept confined to the area where the diarrhea first developed. Wear rubber boots when entering that area and dip them in a disinfection mixture kept in a small tub outside the horse's stall before taking them off. Coveralls for use only in that horse's stall are also a good idea, and be sure to wash your hands immediately after leaving the

stall. Do not walk a horse with diarrhea in the barn. Use separate grooming and feeding equipment. Clean his stall last, preferably with a separate pitchfork and rake. If not using separate cleaning tools, disinfect the ones you use when you are finished. Get a sample of the diarrhea in a clean container for your veterinarian to send for cultures.

When to get veterinary attention:

Veterinary attention is needed immediately if:

- Diarrhea is profuse.
- The horse is not drinking or eating.
- The horse has a temperature over 100° (take temperature three times a day).
- Diarrhea persists for 24 hours.
- Signs of colic develop or worsen.
- Signs of laminitis develop.

Troubleshooting during recovery:

Continue to offer water with electrolytes as well as plain water during recovery. Follow your veterinarian's diet instructions and call if the diarrhea returns.

CONSTIPATION/ IMPACTION ■■

Definition:

Failure to pass manure for several hours

Causes:

- Abnormal intestinal mobility, as with parasite damage
- Change in diet
- Inadequate water intake (most common cause)
- Intestinal blockage by sand, rubber fencing, or an intestinal "stone" (a hard mass of minerals that builds up around a foreign body, known as an enterolith)
- Mechanical blockage such as tumor, abscess, or twisted bowel.

Treatment:

Horse should be evaluated and treated as described under "Colic," page 73.

- One of the most common causes is inadequate water supply or tainted dirty water that the horse does not drink, so offer plenty of clean water.
- Try an electrolyte mixture (see page 79 under "Diarrhea"), in addition to plain water.
- Exercise is helpful with simple constipation.
- If the horse is eating, offer a warm bran mash with one pint of mineral oil added. To make, add two tablespoons of table salt to three to four scoops of bran. Add boiling water to one inch above the level of the bran. Cover with a cloth and allow to sit until all water is absorbed. Thoroughly mix in 1 pint of mineral oil. You may add grated carrots, applesauce, carrot juice, 1/4 cup (maximum) of corn syrup, molasses or dried molasses powder to improve palatability.

When to get veterinary attention:

Call the veterinarian if:

- Constipation persists for 12 hours.
- Signs of colic worsen and do not respond to treatment.
- Signs of laminitis develop.

Troubleshooting during recovery:

After an impaction is relieved, the horse should return to normal. Resolution of impaction may take several days.

WORMS IN THE MANURE ■

This is not a true emergency, but many owners panic if they see worms. Obviously, worms in the manure indicate the horse has a parasite problem. Treatment with a good broad-spectrum dewormer such as Ivermectin is indicated. It is also common to find worms in the manure after the horse has been given a dewormer. This indicates the drug has done its job. If the horse is also showing signs of colic, proceed as above under "Colic," page 73.

08

GRAIN OVERLOAD

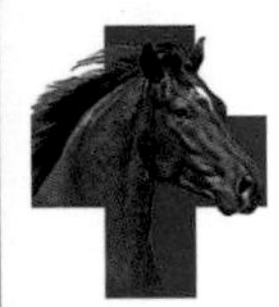

FIRST AID KIT

- Baking soda
- Large (at least 20 cc.) syringe or dose syringe
- Injectable phenylbutazone (for intravenous use only) R_X
- Antihistamine solution (intramuscular injection or oral) R_X
- Analgesics for intramuscular injection – e.g., Banamine or Torbugesic R_X

R_X: PRESCRIPTION DRUG — MUST BE OBTAINED FROM VETERINARIAN OR PRESCRIBED BY A VET — SHOULD NEVER BE ADMINISTERED WITHOUT PRIOR APPROVAL BY A VETERINARIAN.

QUICK CHAPTER REFERENCE LIST

LEGEND: ■■■ — NEEDS EMERGENCY ATTENTION; ■■ — SHOULD BE EXAMINED BY A VET; ■ — MAY NEED VETERINARY ADVICE/ATTENTION

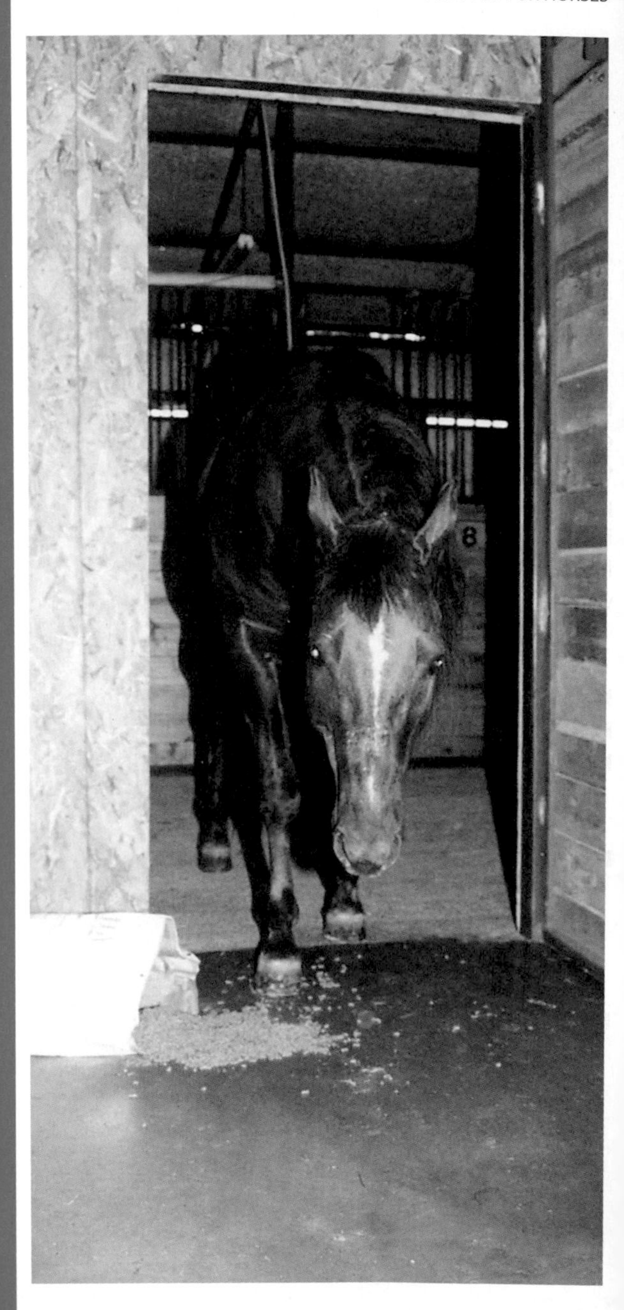
8

GRAIN OVERLOAD

MILD OVERLOAD ■ to ■■

Definition:
Horse has received an extra feeding of grain by mistake or has gotten loose and eaten an amount of grain approximately equal to twice his regular intake.

Symptoms:
Horses will vary from no adverse effects to mild depression and transient loss of appetite to severe problems (listed below under heavy overload). Lameness from laminitis (founder) may appear within the first 24 to 48 hours.

Treatment:

- Withhold all grain for 48 hours.
- Observe the horse for signs of depression.
- Observe him for abdominal distress (sweating, elevated pulse and respiration, looking at or biting flanks, rolling, pawing, loss of appetite, diarrhea).
- Feel the feet hourly for any change in temperature (early laminitis may cause icy cold feet. In the later stages, the feet may feel hotter than usual). Note any lameness or reluctance/refusal to move. (See Chapter 9, page 93)
- If signs of abdominal distress develop, begin monitoring every 15 minutes and consult a veterinarian immediately. If an emergency visit will be delayed, ask the vet about giving 10 teaspoons of baking soda in 20 cc of water (squirt into the back of mouth with a syringe) to counteract acidity. **Never give this or any oral medication to a horse in severe pain and/or obviously bloated.** (Also see "Colic," page 73.

- If temperature changes occur in the horse's feet or if lameness occurs, stand the horse in a slurry of ice and cold water for up to 48 hours, or in a cold running stream if available. Never force the horse to walk or stand if down. Also, the veterinarian may choose to give the horse a nerve block to relieve pain and relieve vascular spasm. After this, the horse will usually be comfortable enough to allow his feet to be picked up and a cushioning layer applied, such as styrofoam or several layers of carpet-ing (see Founder/Laminitis, page 100).
- Avoid oral pain medications (e.g., phenylbutazone) as these cause intestinal tract irritation. By the vet or on the vet's orders only, intravenous pain medications are appropriate (e.g., 2 grams phenylbutazone). Antihistamine therapy early on may be helpful (e.g., tripelennamine or pyrilamine maleate, dose as ordered.) Get veterinary attention.

SEVERE OVERLOAD ■■■

Definition: *Horse had free access to undetermined amount of grain for over 30 minutes or is known to have eaten approximately three times, or more, the usual ration.*

Symptoms: (May see all or some)

- Depression
- Rapid breathing
- Rapid pulse
- Sweating
- Pawing
- Rolling
- Flatulence (passing lots of gas)
- Loss of appetite
- Bloating
- Salivation
- Development of diarrhea (later on)
- Mucous membranes will be bright red to blue-purple in severe cases

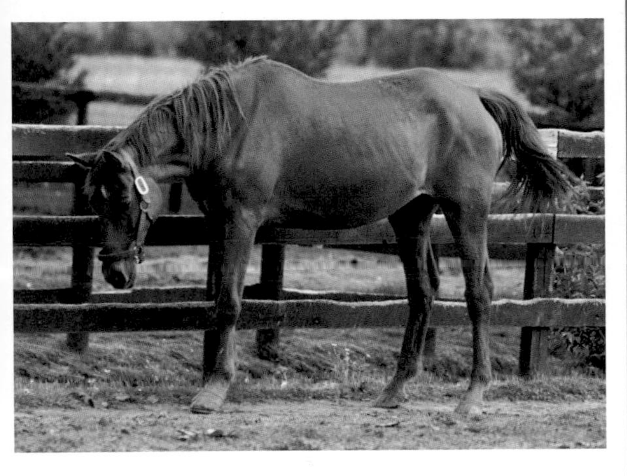

Laminitis flare-ups can cause a horse to stand with his feet out in front of him.

- Sudden, unexplained lessening of pain and obvious bloating, with abnormal mucous membrane color, may signal rupture of stomach.

Complications:
Rupture of stomach; laminitis (founder).

Treatment:

- Call the veterinarian **immediately**.
- Begin recording the horse's symptoms and vital sign and the times you observe them. See page 325 for a helpful form.)
- Remove all hay and water from stall.
- If a veterinarian is not available on an immediate emergency basis, obtain the vet's approval to give 10 teaspoons of baking soda in 20 cc of water for bloating, an obvious distortion of the flanks (behind the ribs and/or lower belly involving one or both sides). **Do not give anything by mouth if the horse is showing signs of severe abdominal pain or bloating.** For pain relief, may give Banamine intramuscularly according to

manufacturer's recommendations, as directed by the vet. The vet might administer Torbugesic.

- Begin icing the feet immediately.

Troubleshooting during recovery:

- Mineral oil will eventually cause the horse to pass loose manure. The manure may also smell foul from fermentation of the extra grain. This should start to revert to more normal manure within 24 hours. If not, call the vet. Charcoal may make the manure look black.
- Laminitis pain should be improving by the third day. It is imperative to get foot X-rays and coordinate with your farrier and vet to get the horse correctly trimmed according to X-ray findings. Failure to do this may cause further damage and will delay recovery.
- Approximately two weeks after an acute laminitis episode, the horse may appear to worsen. This is usually due to collections of serum and blood in the feet trying to come to the surface and "abscess" through. Do **not** give pain relievers or anti-inflammatory drugs. These will slow or block the drainage/abscessation process. Consult your vet about the advisability of soaking or other procedures.

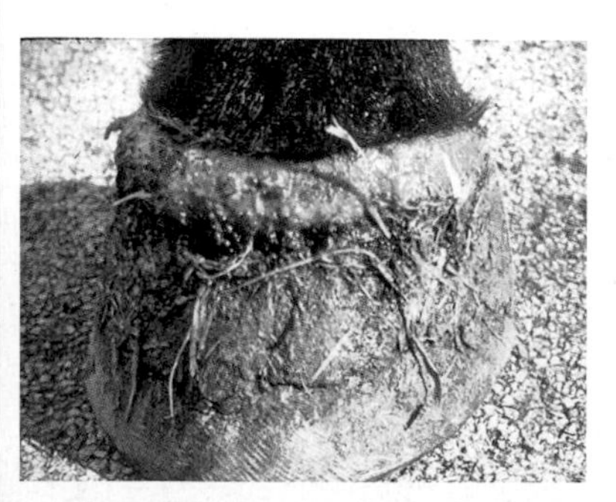

Coronitis, inflammation of the coronary band, can be seen with laminitis or contact with irritant substances.

09
LAMENESS

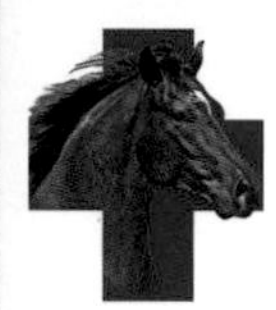

FIRST AID KIT

- Large sterile gauze pads
- Iodine solution
- Hydrogen peroxide
- Xylazine (Rompun) ℞
- Acepromazine ℞
- Foot packing or poultice
- Alcohol (rubbing or isopropyl)
- Mild liniment
- Phenylbutazone ℞
- Elastic self-adherent wrap, such as Vetrap
- Bandages
- Roll cotton or thick leg wraps
- Thick carpet or styrofoam

℞: PRESCRIPTION DRUG — MUST BE OBTAINED FROM VETERINARIAN OR PRESCRIBED BY A VET — SHOULD NEVER BE ADMINISTERED WITHOUT PRIOR APPROVAL BY A VETERINARIAN.

QUICK CHAPTER REFERENCE LIST

LEGEND: ■■■ — NEEDS EMERGENCY ATTENTION; ■■ — SHOULD BE EXAMINED BY A VET; ■ — MAY NEED VETERINARY ADVICE/ATTENTION

LAMENESS

DEGREES OF LAMENESS

Lameness is described as:
- 1° (slight)
- 2° (easily visible)
- 3° (total inability or refusal to bear weight).

Only 3° lameness can be considered an emergency. This chapter will deal with 2° and 3° lameness.

Symptoms of lameness:
- Limping
- Shortened stride length
- Reluctance to work on a circle in the direction of the lame leg
- Resting or pointing the lame leg at rest
- Rough gaits
- Change in performance (e.g., change in jumping style) and/or development of an uncooperative attitude toward work.

There are specific signs that relate to particular areas, such as swinging the leg to the outside with knee pain, but a full description of these is outside the scope of this book and is best left to the veterinarian examining the horse.

Diagnosis:
In general, the horse will take shorter strides with his lame leg and come down harder on the opposite leg. His

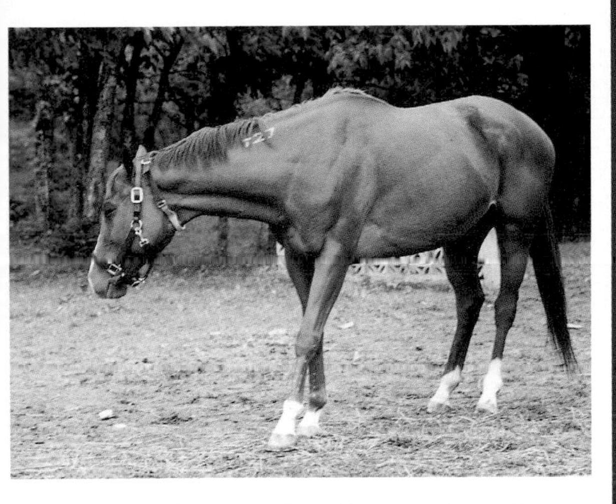

A horse with severe foot pain may be unable to put weight on the affected foot.

head will drop when placing weight on the good leg and will jerk up on the bad side; this is known as "nodding." Also, when viewed from in front or behind, the horse may move the painful leg in an abnormal manner, swinging it in or out, placing it further under his body when the foot lands, or any other deviation from bringing the leg forward smoothly in a straight line. Lameness is usually more obvious when the horse is worked on hard ground.

Once you feel you have located the sore leg, examination of the leg will help to locate the problem. The three cardinal signs of inflammation are swelling, heat, and pain. Begin at the foot and work your way up the leg, comparing the temperature and any amount of swelling with the opposite leg. Pain may be evident when you press an area or, if a joint, when the leg is picked up and the joint flexed. Holding the joint flexed for 30 to 60 seconds and then immediately jogging the horse off will usually cause the lameness to worsen.

Treatment:

2° Lameness ■■: Acute injuries, or flare-ups of old problems, may respond to aggressive anti-inflammatory therapy. Hose the affected area with cold water (or soak in a bucket of cold water) for 15 to 20 minutes, three to four times daily. If the problem is in the foot, keep the foot packed with either poultice or a hoof packing. Problems in the fetlock (ankles), cannon bones, splints or tendons/ligaments below the knees may benefit from wrapping the leg between hosings. Massage the leg with alcohol or a cooling liniment for 5 to 10 minutes before wrapping. The massage should also be done for problems higher on the leg that cannot be wrapped. The above procedures should be done for three days.

The horse can also be placed on a three-day course of anti-inflammatory drug therapy with 1 to 2 grams of phenylbutazone paste or powder given by mouth, once or twice daily (dosage is for adult, 1,000-pound horses). On the fourth day, discontinue water therapy and phenylbutazone but continue massage and wrapping. Begin hand walking the horse, with a gradual return to work if he stays sound.

When to call the veterinarian:

- If the location of the lameness cannot be determined.
- If the lameness worsens.
- If the lameness fails to improve after three days of treatment as listed above.
- If the lameness returns a day or so after phenylbutazone is stopped.

3° Lameness ■■: When a horse refuses to bear weight, or only minimally touches the ground with the involved leg, emergency veterinary attention is indicated. Don't give large doses of phenylbutazone until the horse has been evaluated by the vet. However, if pain and distress

Which leg is lame?

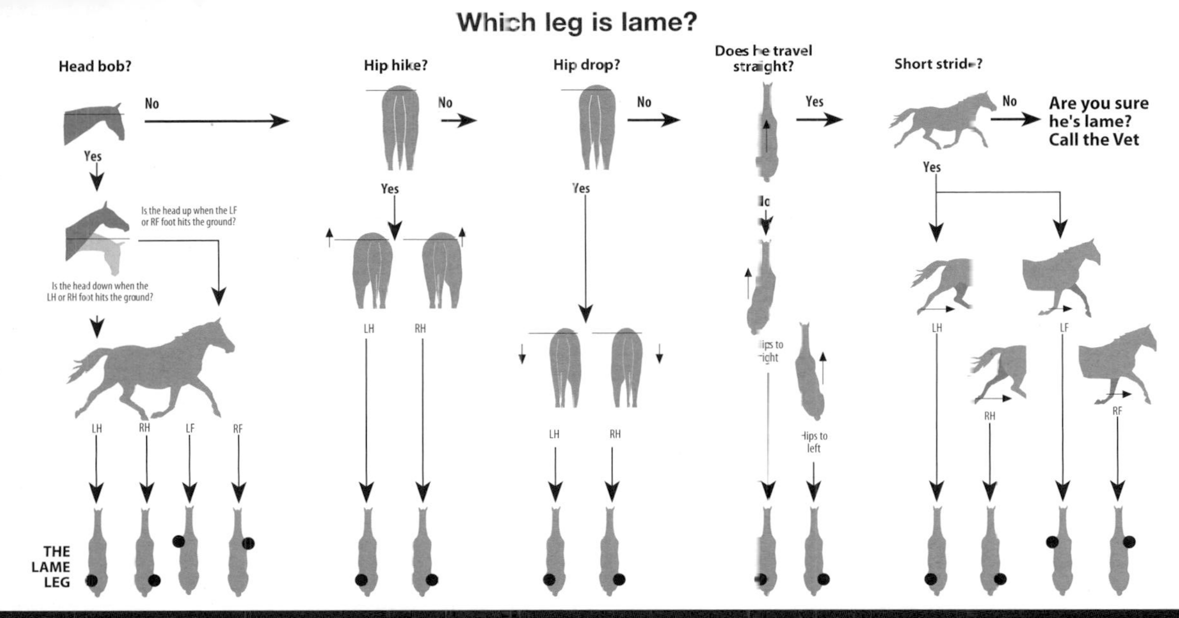

© ILLUSTRATED BY KIP CARTER

are severe, you may give 1 to 2 grams of phenylbutazone with the vet's approval. The opposite leg, which is taking an increased load, should be wrapped to provide support. If possible the foot of the "good" leg should be packed with poultice or hoof packing to provide additional support. (Founder in the "good" leg is a common complication of severe lameness.) Check packing frequently and replace it if it starts to dry out.

TENDON/LIGAMENT INJURIES ■■■

The horse has two flexor tendons (deep and superficial flexor) and a suspensory ligament running behind the cannon bone in the lower leg. These are fairly common sites of injury that can range from a simple strain/sprain with no actual damage to the fibers, to a complete rupture. Signs of the problem may show up either immediately after work, or may take a day or two to be obvious. The area will be swollen and feel hot to the touch.

The degree of lameness is variable but it usually correlates with how severe the injury is — i.e., if horse is very lame, injury is likely severe. Rupture will cause the fetlock (ankle) to drop down lower than normal when the horse puts weight on the injured leg, but there may be enough pain that the horse is not willing to put much, if any, weight on the leg.

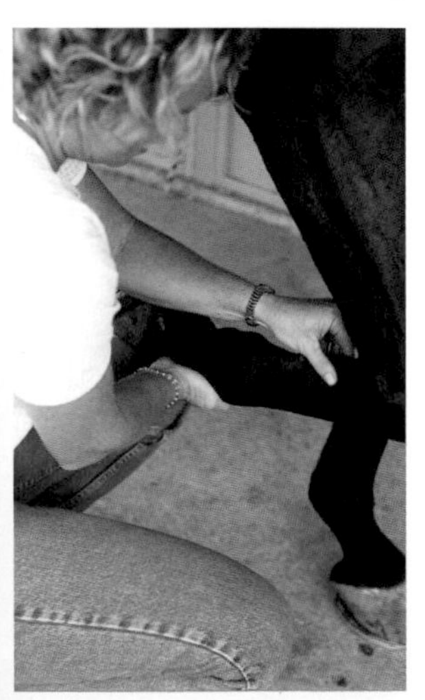

When the horse is lame, feel his legs from the feet up, checking for heat, swelling or tenderness.

Swelling in the lower portion of flexor tendon.

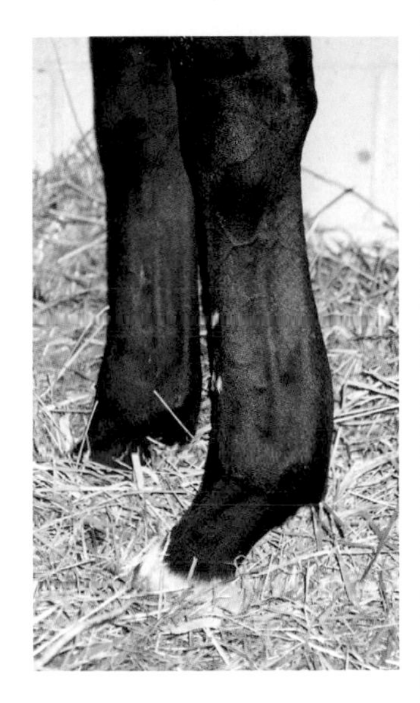

Emergency treatment is as on page 96 for 3° lameness. The leg should be wrapped between cooling treatments, but this must be done by someone who is experienced with wrapping damaged tendons and ligaments, since too much pressure or uneven pressure may cause more damage. If the horse's fetlock is dropping down closer to the ground than a normal position, or if the lameness is severe, get immediate veterinary attention. Otherwise, if the swelling and pain take longer than 24 hours to resolve, an ultrasound examination should be done to determine the degree of damage and proper amount of rest needed before working the horse again.

Troubleshooting during recovery:

- When the horse is on rest, swelling and heat should steadily diminish. Alert the vet if either doesn't.
- When the horse resumes gradual exercise, minor flare ups of swelling and heat may occur as a natural part of the remodeling process. These should respond within 24 hours to icing and wrapping. If not, alert your vet.
- Resume the exercise process slowly.

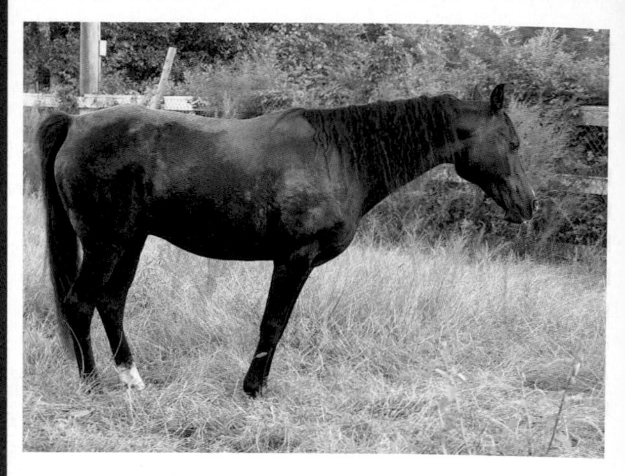

This horse is a rare instance of active laminitis worse in the hind limbs. The sweating is due to pain.

FOUNDER/LAMINITIS ■■■

Also see Chapter 8, on Grain Overload, page 85.

Laminitis is a breakdown of the attachments between the coffin bone inside the hoof and the hoof wall. It is a medical emergency that requires prompt veterinary treatment to avoid serious damage to the feet.

Symptoms include:

- Depression, elevated pulse and elevated respiratory rate caused by pain.
- Reluctance or absolute refusal to move.
- Standing with the front feet either farther in front of the body than normal, or farther underneath it.
- Pounding pulses behind the ankle, over the sesamoid bones.
- Feet feel hot to the touch.

Front feet are usually more affected than rear. Laminitis must be suspected in any horse showing reluctance to move for an unclear reason. Fracture or abscess inside the foot may also cause this degree of lameness, but will rarely involve both feet.

Treatment:

- Call the vet immediately.
- Call the farrier.
- Do **not** force the horse to move.
- If no cause is obvious, the root may be metabolic. Remove from pasture. Feed only soaked grass hay. No grain, balancers, carrots or other treats. Do not bed on straw.
- If the vet will be delayed in arriving and you have it on hand, ask about administering phenylbutazone (2 to 3 grams/1,000 pound horse) and acepromazine (tranquilizer and vasodilator, 10 mg per 1,000-pound horse).
- If the feet can be picked up, tape on several layers of carpeting or thick Styrofoam, cut to the size of the foot.

Troubleshooting during recovery:
Drainage of abscesses (pus, old blood, or serum) should be expected during recovery. This is a good thing, and release of this material will make the horse more comfortable. Complete recovery requires:

- Frequent trims or shoe resets. May be required as often as every 2 to 3 weeks to keep the foot properly trimmed and balanced.
- Underlying cause must be identified and corrected.
- Formal exercise, especially with a rider, should be avoided until the horse has grown a completely new hoof (6 to 12 months depending on the horse).
- Failure to do these things may cause another flare up of the laminitis, and more damage to the foot. If the horse is experiencing an obvious worsening of pain, consult the vet immediately.

FRACTURE ■■■

Closed fractures: Bone not exposed. Fracture should always be suspected in horses that are 3° lame. In many cases, the fracture will be obvious, with extensive heat, swelling, and pain; dangling of the leg below the fracture or abnormal movement of the fractured area. You may also be able to feel pieces of bone just under the skin.

Treatment:

- Call for veterinary help immediately.
- For emergency treatment before the vet arrives, give a large dose of phenylbutazone (three to four grams for a 1,000-pound adult horse) preferably intravenously if you are experienced at IV injections and the vet approves. If it must be given orally, use a paste preparation or mix the crushed powder with corn syrup or heavy molasses and place it on back of the horse's tongue. Allow 30 minutes for full analgesic effect.

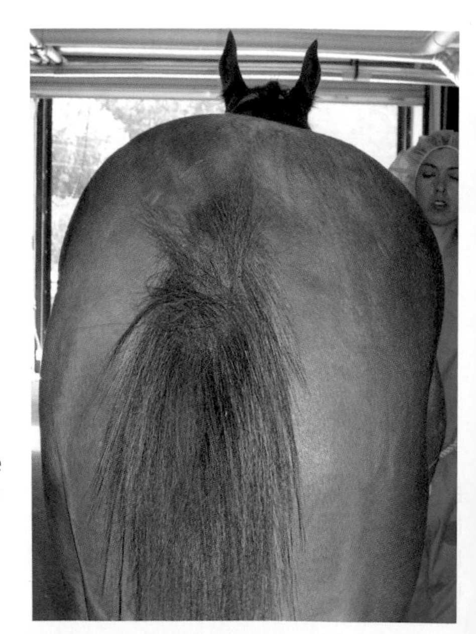

When there is an obvious difference from side to side in the height of the point of the rump, with the horse standing with hind legs even, a pelvic problem is likely.

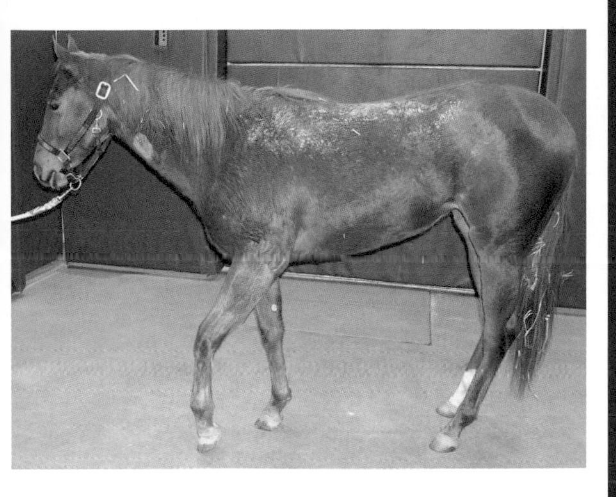

With this elbow fracture, the horse is not able to bear weight on the left front.

- If the horse is extremely agitated, moving around a great deal or generally resisting attempts at treatment, he should be tranquilized. However, sedation may worsen unsteadiness in a horse that has sustained the shock of a fracture. Give the horse 10 to 15 minutes in quiet, familiar surroundings before beginning any emergency treatment. **Do not tranquilize without approval from the vet.** Rompun is the tranquilizer of choice as it will also give you about 15 minutes of analgesic effect. Give intramuscularly or intravenously at 0.125 mg/lb. dose initially, repeating this in 20 minutes if not adequate. Allow 10 to 15 minutes after giving this drug to evaluate its effect. Sedation may be very profound, as the horse has been severely stressed by the severe injury.

Be prepared to work on the horse where he is, as moving him is dangerous in terms of the fracture and because of the sedation. To begin, place a good support bandage on the opposite leg (packing the foot will not be possible). Have an assistant gently hold the fractured leg in as close to a normal position as possible, without undue manipulation of the bones. Wrap the involved area with several thick layers of cotton, followed by a self-adhesive wrap, such as Vetrap. If available, incorporate two pieces of light wood, cork or plastic into the bandage, placing these on top of the cotton and under the elastic wrap. These should extend several inches above and below the fracture site. Use the lightest splint material possible, as the weight of this might tend to make the bandage slip down. If it seems safe to walk the horse, proceed very slowly to the closest stall and place him in extra bedding. Allow the horse to lie down if he insists on doing so. However it is best to keep him standing until the veterinarian arrives. See emergency splints, Chapter 26, page 287.

Open fractures: An open fracture is one where bone is protruding through the skin. This is a very serious condition, as infected bone heals poorly and is very difficult to treat.

Treatment:

- Call the vet and give tranquilizer and pain relief therapy as described above, as approved by the vet.
- Clean the area by first running cold water over it (direct the water stream above the fracture, not into it) for 15 to 20 minutes. This will control inflammation and pain and help to wash out any debris. Do not attempt to directly clean the fracture area or touch it in any way.
- After hosing, pour hydrogen peroxide over the wound, again directing it above the fracture and allowing it to run down over it, until the entire surface is "fizzing" white. Leave this on while you gently remove as much dirt and blood surrounding the wound as you can without unduly disturbing the horse.

- Finally, rinse off the peroxide with cold water. If heavy bleeding is interfering with these procedures, see Chapter 5, page 48.

After the wound has been cleaned and bleeding is controlled, cover the area with gauze or linen (no cotton or other material with loose fibers) soaked in iodine solution. Carefully proceed with bandaging as described above for closed fractures, making certain the iodine-soaked bandage does not become displaced, exposing the wound to cotton. Keep the horse on his feet until the vet arrives. You may give tetanus antitoxin/toxoid if on hand, and antibiotics, but consult with the veterinarian first.

Troubleshooting during recovery:
Return of severe pain after work is resumed should be evaluated by the vet, as it may mean re-fracture. However, low level "lameness" at this time may be due to the injured leg being weak and not as well muscled. If the horse doesn't begin to move better after a few weeks of a careful exercise or turnout, get advice regarding appropriate exercises or modifications of work.

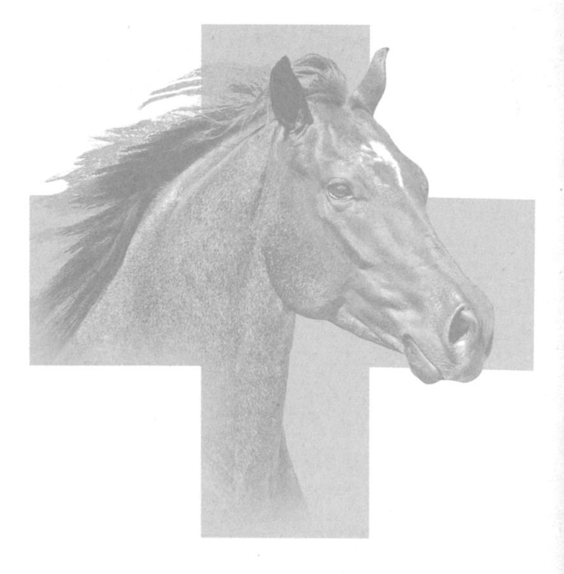

10

HEAT STROKE

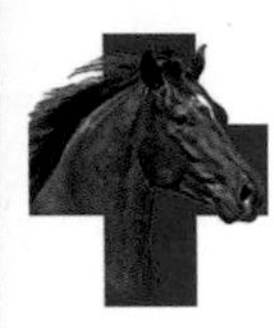

FIRST AID KIT

- Ice
- Sodium chloride (table salt)
- Potassium chloride (salt substitute)
- Bicarbonate (baking soda)
- Thermometer

QUICK CHAPTER REFERENCE LIST

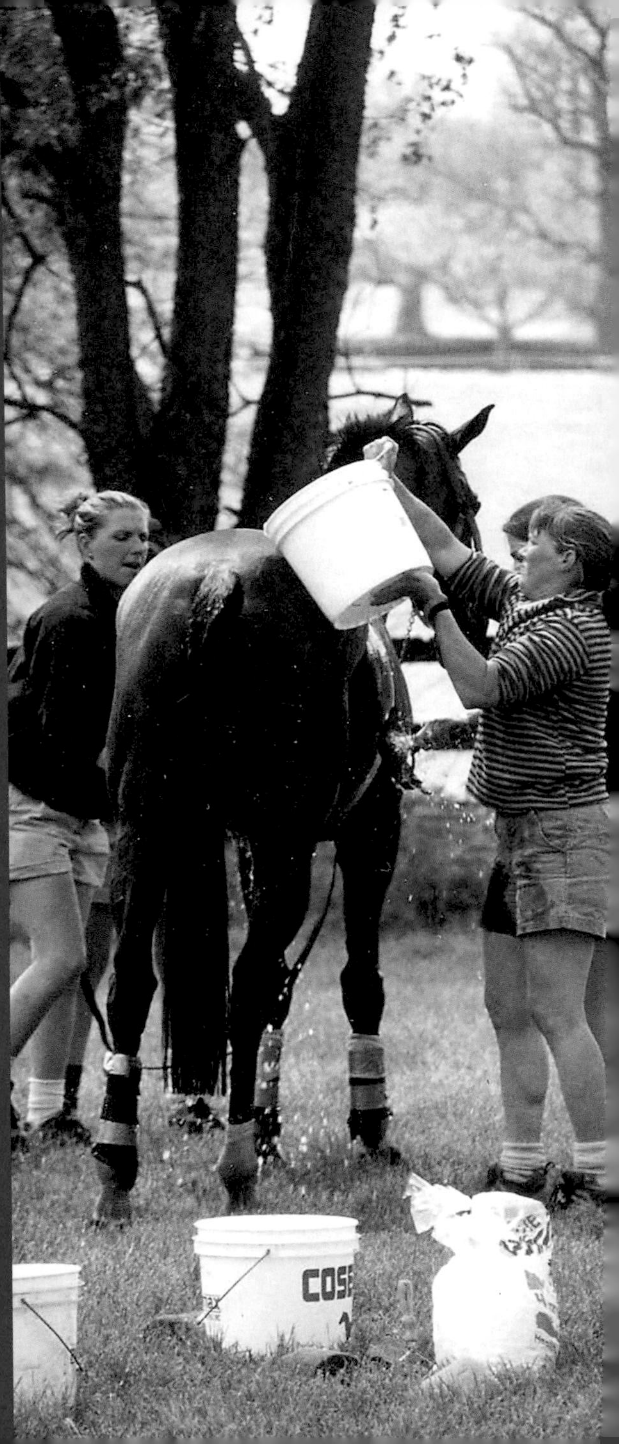

HEAT STROKE

HEAT STROKE ■■■

Definition: *Heat stroke, heat exhaustion, and sun stroke refer to a disturbance of the heat-regulating mechanisms of the body. This is usually associated with exercise in extreme heat, but it may also occur in animals left in direct sun with no access to water. An inadequate salt supply may increase the susceptibility to heat stroke, as can hard work for several days in a row in hot weather or the use of diuretics.*

Symptoms:
- Muscular cramping
- Profound weakness or collapse
- Muscle tremors
- Profuse sweating
- No sweating despite the heat
- Rapid breathing
- Rapid pulse.

Working animals may refuse to go further and drop in their tracks. Rectal body temperature may be greatly elevated (up to 109°F or greater). Mucous membranes are brick red. The horse may also stare as if in a daze and be unresponsive.

Treatment:
The primary goal of treatment must be to lower the horse's body temperature.
- Hose the animal with cold water continuously until his temperature returns to normal.

- Place ice packs around his body and between the legs if the horse is lying down.
- The rectum may be packed with cracked ice, but this removes the possibility of monitoring temperature to determine effectiveness of therapy. There is also the possibility of causing damage to the rectum, resulting in life-threatening infection in the abdomen. In general, while ice in the rectum is highly effective, its use should be withheld for cases where the temperature remains extremely high despite other measures. (You may try positioning the thermometer for an oral reading if the animal doesn't object; oral temperature will be at least one degree lower than rectal.)
- Veterinary aid should be obtained as quickly as possible to administer intravenous fluids, preferably cooled fluids. Animals willing to drink should be offered their choice of both fresh water and electrolyte water. (Use a commercial mix or add 1 ounce table salt, 1 ounce salt substitute [potassium chloride] and 5 tablespoons of baking soda to 5 gallons of water.) Increase the table salt to 2 ounces if baking soda is not available.
- Horses that are willing to stand and move should be transported to a cool and shady area. Prostrate horses should not be moved. A temporary shade should be erected over them, with only a top so the air can circulate.

Troubleshooting during recovery:
Emergency vet treatments may not completely reverse dehydration. The horse should have easy access to both plain water and water with salt added during recovery. Problems that may occur over the next 24 hours include colic from altered gut motility or disruption of the gut micro-organisms, or kidney damage if the muscles have been severely injured and have released a large load of pigment (myoglobin). Observe the horse carefully to make sure he's eating, urinating, and passing manure normally.

11

EXERCISE-RELATED PROBLEMS

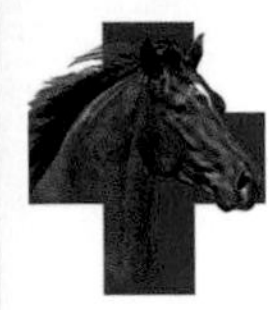

FIRST AID KIT

- Sodium chloride (table salt)
- Potassium chloride (salt substitute)
- Bicarbonate (baking soda)
- Acepromazine ℞
- Phenylbutazone ℞
- Banamine ℞

℞: PRESCRIPTION DRUG — MUST BE OBTAINED FROM VETERINARIAN OR PRESCRIBED BY A VET — SHOULD NEVER BE ADMINISTERED WITHOUT PRIOR APPROVAL BY A VETERINARIAN.

QUICK CHAPTER REFERENCE LIST

LEGEND: ■■■ — NEEDS EMERGENCY ATTENTION; ■■ — SHOULD BE EXAMINED BY A VET;
■ — MAY NEED VETERINARY ADVICE/ATTENTION

EXERCISE-RELATED PROBLEMS

EXHAUSTION/HEAT PROSTRATION ■■■

Symptoms:

- Marked depression after exercise
- Loss of appetite
- Refusal to drink
- Continued sweating
- Elevated pulse
- Temperature
- Respiratory rates beyond 15 to 20 minutes post-exercise.

Cause:

Overwork.

Treatment:

See Chapter 10, on Heat Stroke, page 109. Make certain the horse has free access to water and salt after being cooled out.

THUMPS ■■

Definition:

Thumps is a condition of severe electrolyte disturbances in which the diaphragm is stimulated to move synchronously with the heart beat.

Symptoms:

A jerking to heavy thumping movement behind the last rib, in the flank, occurring in a horse with one or more symptoms of overwork. Appears like hiccups.

Treatment:

Calcium, potassium, and magnesium are the primary electrolyte disturbances responsible for the problem, together with dehydration and alterations in pH and chloride content of the blood.

- Cool the horse out.
- Offer him both plain water and water with electrolytes, and allow him to eat.
- If the symptoms do not disappear after eating and drinking and/or within two to three hours, the horse will require specialized electrolyte mixtures given by the veterinarian intravenously.

TYING UP ■■ to ■■■

Definition:

Severe and persistent muscular cramping that occurs during or immediately after exercise or some excitement.

Symptoms:

- Extreme anxiety and/or depression
- Elevated pulse and respiratory rates (secondary to pain)
- Reluctance or refusal to move
- Rigid stance
- Rock-hard musculature, primarily in the large muscles of the hindquarters
- Dark urine.

What to do:

- Move the horse as little as possible. Forced exercise — even walking — can cause more muscle breakdown.
- If the horse has been competing or exercising some distance from the barn, trailer him back to the barn.
- If the weather is cool, blanket the horse and protect him from drafts.
- Offer both fresh and electrolyte water (see chapter 10, page 112).
- After clearance from the vet, give 20 to 30 mg. of Acepromazine tranquilizer intramuscularly. For a 1,000-

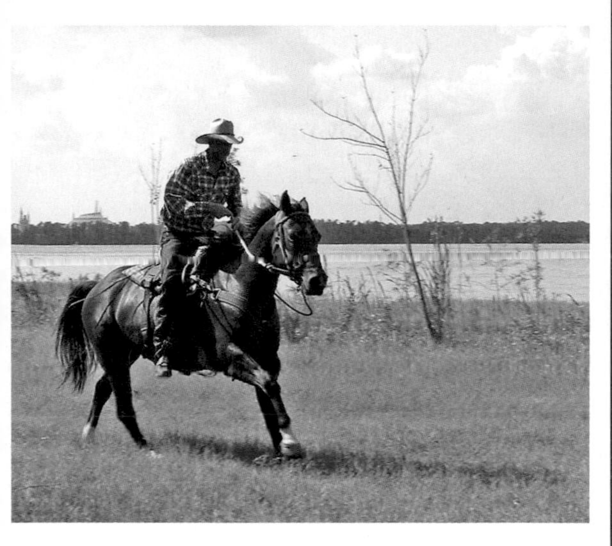

True tying up is always precipitated by exercise, or in some rare cases by shipping. Tying up is a medical emergency.

pound horse, give 2 to 3 grams of phenylbutazone paste or slurry (or intravenous injection) or 500 mg. of Banamine for pain and inflammation.

- Observe the urine carefully. Dark urine indicates the presence of muscle pigment, a severe sign. If urine color is not clear by the second time the horse urinates, get immediate veterinary attention, as the muscle pigment can plug the kidneys and cause renal failure.

When to call the veterinarian:

- If the urine remains dark on two separate urinations.
- If the horse's condition is not improved after the drug therapy recommended above.
- If the horse refuses all water for more than one hour.

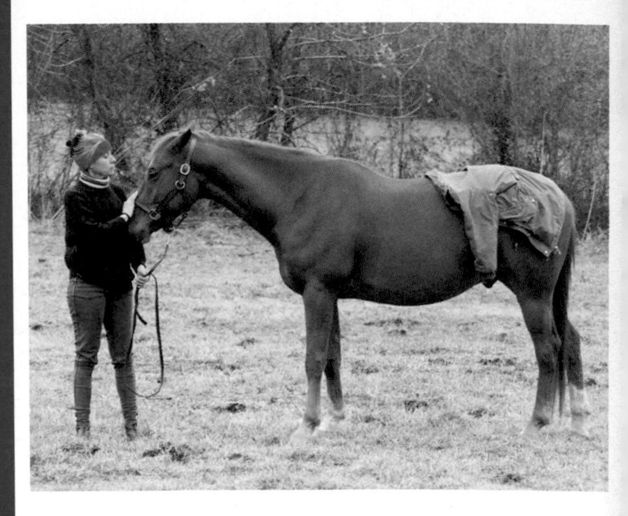

Do not force a horse that is "tying up" to move. Cover him with a sheet, cooler or heavy blanket, depending on the weather conditions, and call the vet immediately.

Conditions that may be confused with tying up:

- Laminitis.
- Coffin-bone fractures.
- Severe chest pain.
- Severe abdominal pain.
- Tetanus.

All of the above can cause the horse to be reluctant to move, stand stiffly, and shift his weight to the hindquarters, making the hind-end muscles tense up.

If you find the horse with symptoms that look like tying up but there has been no exercise, it's not tying up.

12

BREATHING PROBLEMS

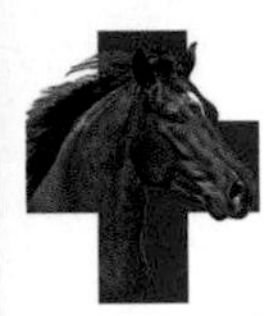

FIRST AID KIT

- Thermometer
- Vicks VapoRub
- Blanket
- Phenylbutazone ℞
- Cough suppressant recommended by veterinarian
- Vaporizer
- Expectorant recommended by veterinarian (e.g., sodium iodide powder)
- Vaseline
- Scalpel and emergency breathing tube (for tracheostomy)
- Gauze pads
- Antibiotics ℞
- Tranquilizer ℞
- Tetanus antitoxin and toxoid ℞

℞: PRESCRIPTION DRUG — MUST BE OBTAINED FROM VETERINARIAN OR PRESCRIBED BY A VET — SHOULD NEVER BE ADMINISTERED WITHOUT PRIOR APPROVAL BY A VETERINARIAN.

QUICK CHAPTER REFERENCE LIST

LEGEND: ■■■ — NEEDS EMERGENCY ATTENTION; ■■ — SHOULD BE EXAMINED BY A VET;
■ — MAY NEED VETERINARY ADVICE/ATTENTION

BREATHING PROBLEMS

RAPID RESPIRATION

■ to ■■■

Definition:
A respiratory rate of over 15 breaths per minute is considered rapid in an adult horse.

Nonspecific causes:
Pain, fear, exercise

Respiratory causes:
- Infection of the lungs or chest (check for one or more of the respiratory symptoms listed below in this chapter).
- Allergy

Treatment:
- Count and write down the number of breaths per minute.
- Blanket the horse if the weather dictates, and keep him out of drafts.
- Check for and write down any other symptoms.
- Take his temperature.
- Contact the veterinarian with the above information.
- Get emergency attention if the horse's breathing is obviously difficult and he is agitated or depressed.

NOISY RESPIRATION

■ to ■■■

Definition:
Any noise that occurs with breathing (normal respiration is silent).

Nonspecific causes:
Pain may cause the horse to make blowing or grunting noises.

Respiratory causes:

- Anatomical abnormalities along the upper airways (nose and throat) can block the normal flow of air and cause noisy breathing.
- Swelling anywhere along the upper airways or windpipe (e.g., from trauma, infection, or allergic reaction) does the same thing.
- Infections in the lungs may cause excessive secretions that obstruct air flow.

Types of Noises:

- **Blowing:** Forceful, hard breathing, as occurs after exercise or if the horse is in pain.
- **Wheezing:** High-pitched, squeaking noises that are usually most obvious when the horse exhales.
- **Whistling:** High-pitched, fluttering or flute-like noises, usually more obvious during one phase of respiration (i.e., either when breathing out or breathing in).
- **Rattling:** Coarse, wet or dry noises that are heard throughout respiration, associated with collection of fluid or mucus along the respiratory tract.

Causes and what to do:

Blowing: Blowing after exercise is normal. Depending on the exercise, it lasts from a few minutes to 20 minutes. If the horse does not recover after 20 minutes, take his temperature. Walk the horse to check for signs of lameness or reluctance to move that might indicate a source of pain. If the horse is overheated (temperature over 100° after 20 minutes), sponge or hose him with lukewarm water. If no other cause is found, schedule a veterinary examination to check for breathing problems.

If the horse is blowing without relation to exercise, the cause is usually moderate to severe pain. Fever may also cause blowing, so take the horse's temperature. Try to determine the cause of pain by walking the horse and checking his stall for anything abnormal (e.g., change in or lack of manure). Seek emergency attention and treatment.

Wheezing: Wheezing may be caused by allergic/asthma-type reactions ("heaves") or accumulation of dry mucus in the lungs during or after a respiratory infection. Exercise may worsen wheezing to the point where you can hear it without a stethoscope. If there is no history of infections, the horse may be relieved by taking him outside, since most irritants are found in the barn — hay and straw. If the wheezing does not stop or if the horse is depressed and working hard to breathe, emergency attention is needed. Otherwise, schedule a visit for evaluation and recommendations for medication and management.

Whistling: Whistling noises associated with exercise, excitement, or any elevated breathing rate usually signal a structural problem in the upper airways (e.g., "roaring," growths, cysts, or other problem). The noise will abate if the horse is kept quiet, but diagnosis and treatment will eventually be necessary. If whistling appears suddenly, is not associated with exercise, and does not go away when the horse is kept quiet, seek emergency attention. The cause is likely to be a sudden blockage to breathing from an abscess, tumor, or collection of infections somewhere. Check the throat area (between jaw bones) for swelling or drainage of pus, which is likely to be "Strangles" infection. Take the horse's temperature and get immediate attention.

Rattling: Rattling noises, as already stated, accompany collections of fluid or mucus along the respiratory tract. Take the horse's temperature and note any other symptoms (e.g., cough or nasal discharge). Keep the horse quiet and warm. Liberal use of Vicks VapoRub and a vaporizer will help to loosen the secretions. Do not start antibiotics without consulting the vet since antibiotics will interfere with any necessary cultures. For temperature over 100°, depression, loss of appetite or obvious difficulty in breathing, seek emergency attention.

Troubleshooting:
If the breathing does not improve within 24 hours of starting the vet-recommended treatment, or if it worsens at any time, call the vet.

FLARED NOSTRILS ■■

Definition:
Nostrils blown wide open with each breath, usually accompanied by blowing (see above).

Causes:
Flaring is associated with hard breathing of any cause. It is a sign that the horse is working hard to get air. This is normal for a short period after exercise, but at other times indicates the horse has a problem with getting enough air. On occasion, the hard breathing associated with severe pain will also cause flaring.

Treatment:
Flaring not associated with exercise indicates the horse is not getting sufficient air. Take his temperature, avoid all stress (do not move the horse), protect him from cold and drafts, record any other symptoms, and get emergency attention.

COUGH ■ to ■■■

Causes and what to do:
Cough is caused by any irritation (infection or otherwise) along the respiratory tract.

Dry Cough: Caused by early viral infections or irritation from dust/allergens. Take the horse's temperature three times daily. If fever is present, suspect probable early viral infection.

- Watch for nasal discharge (clear with uncomplicated virus, yellow or grey with bacterial infection).
- Avoid cold and drafts, and keep the horse in a stall until his temperature is normal for 24 hours.
- Encourage eating with high-quality hay and mashes.
- Avoid all medications unless absolutely necessary.

With constant cough, you may give an over-the-counter equine cough medicine for a day or two. If the cough persists, call your vet. If fever (over 100°) is present on two consecutive readings, you may give 1 to 2 grams phenylbutazone per 1,000 pounds once a day, but not for more than two days. If fever persists at high levels, if the cough is severe, if there is a white-yellow or grey discharge, or if any other respiratory symptoms listed in this chapter are severe, get veterinary attention. Do not give antibiotics without consulting a vet. The horse and his equipment should be isolated from other animals, since respiratory infections are highly contagious.

If there is no fever or other sign of infection, the probable cause of a dry cough is allergy ("heaves"). For a severe attack, get immediate attention. Otherwise, put the horse outside, and feed only clean, dust-free hay and grain. Consult a veterinarian if the problem persists.

Moist Cough: A wet cough is almost always associated with respiratory infection — either a complication of viral infection or following allergic irritation. Nasal discharge may not be visible if the horse is swallowing his secretions.

- Avoid cold and drafts.
- No exercise.
- Keep secretions loose with a vaporizer and Vicks in the nose.
- If these measures do not provide relief in a day, or if the horse is not getting any better, call a vet.
- Do not give antibiotics without consulting a veterinarian.
- Do not give cough suppressants when a moist cough is present.

NASAL DISCHARGE

■ to ■■■

Definition:
Fluid from the nostrils.

Causes:

Mechanical irritation or infection. Cold weather alone causes some horses to have a constant clear discharge. A clear to frothy-white discharge is also common after hard exercise or in cold weather and is not necessarily a cause for concern .

Danger signs include:

- Heavy discharge associated with abnormal breathing.
- Yellowish, grayish, thick discharge.
- Discharge from one side only caused by infection or structural problem in the nasal passages, sinuses, or throat).

Treatment:

- Seek immediate veterinary attention if the horse is having trouble breathing.
- Schedule an examination to find the cause if the horse is not in immediate distress.

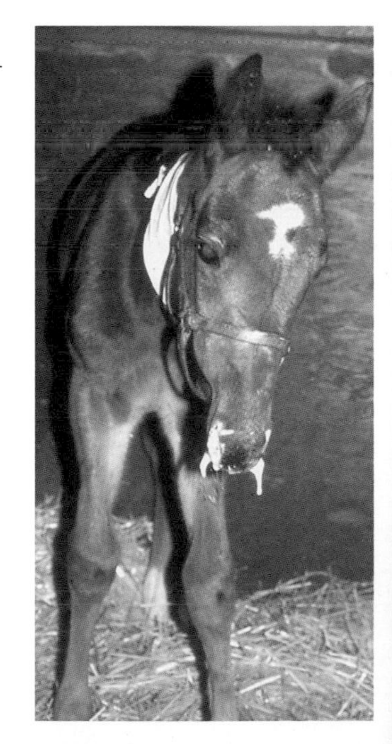

Call the vet if you see a heavy, white discharge.

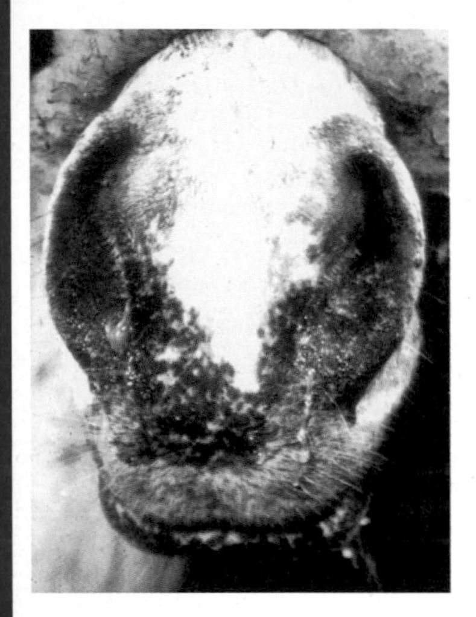

Pus from the nostrils indicates a serious infection.

- Take his temperature 2 to 3 times daily.
- Record all other symptoms.
- Do not give antibiotics without veterinary approval.
- Keep his nostrils wiped clean and coated with Vaseline to avoid skin irritation.

Troubleshooting:
If his breathing does not improve within 24 hours of starting the vet-recommended treatment, or if it worsens at any time, call the vet.

Reducing risk of respiratory infections:
- Very young (3 and under) or old horses are the most susceptible to respiratory infections.
- Your best protection against a serious respiratory infection is a healthy horse with a strong immune system.
- Vaccinations provide incomplete protection, at best, but can help reduce severity of symptoms and reduce the number of infectious organisms shed. Always vaccinate well in advance (at least 2 weeks) of high-risk periods. Talk to your vet about a vaccination schedule

prior to cold weather, paying special attention to horses that travel extensively, or are exposed to horses frequently coming and going from their environment.

- During an outbreak, **keep all infected horses and those that have been in direct contact with infected horses away from direct contact with healthy horses.** If possible, keep healthy horses in another building or even outside. Use separate buckets, brushes, etc. for the infected and healthy horses. Wash your hands between horses. Ventilate the barn well, but avoid direct drafts. Take temperatures twice daily of horses that appear well. Immediately quarantine horses that develop temperatures above 101° or have other symptoms.
- May vaccinate horses that remain well only if they have been without temperature elevation or other symptoms for 10 days after the start of the outbreak. (If the horse is incubating the disease, vaccination may result in illness.)

BLEEDING FROM NOSE See Chapter 5, page 50.

TRAUMA TO NECK/THROAT ■■ to ■■■

An injury to the neck or throat area should be evaluated to determine if it needs veterinary attention (see Chapter 4, page 27 and Chapter 15, page 153). If a horse with a neck wound is making abnormal breathing sounds, get veterinary help immediately. If the horse has suffered a severe blow or crushing-type injury to the throat or neck area and is having trouble breathing, (even though the skin is not broken), he has crushed or fractured a part of his respiratory tract or is having his air choked off by severe swelling or bleeding into the tissues. Call for emergency attention and keep the horse as quiet as possible. **Never tranquilize a horse having breathing problems — this may depress breathing further.**

Emergency tracheostomy

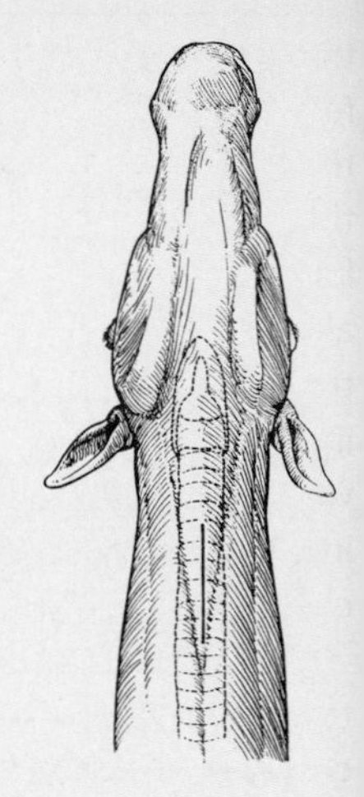

If the horse has a wound in the windpipe area, you're going to work with that opening to help the horse get air. If not, you'll have to make an opening.

Once the horse has collapsed (from lack of oxygen), immediately locate the windpipe. Try to find an opening into the windpipe from the injury, assuming that it's at least 6 inches down the neck, away from the horse's throat. (If you cannot find an opening into the trachea, you'll have to make one. see below.) Spread this open as widely as possible and push aside any muscle or other tissue that might be in the way.

Ideally you will need to place something in the opening from the injury to keep it open. The outside cylinder of a 20 cc syringe (with the nozzle end cut off) is a good size for this. (If you cannot get a 20 cc syringe barrel to fit without putting excessive pressure on the hard, cartilage "rings" of the trachea, use a 12 cc syringe.) It should be positioned perpendicular to the windpipe on top of the throat so that it does not fall down into the windpipe.

If the horse does not have a wound near the windpipe and at least 6 inches down the neck from the throat, you will need to make an incision through the skin over the trachea. Feel for the windpipe through the skin, about 4 to 5 inches below throat level. Feel for the tracheal rings, which feel like ridges. Pull the skin tight over the trachea with one hand and cut boldly all the way through the skin and underlying tissues. Don't worry about bleeding at this point. Don't worry about cutting into the trachea. It is very tough and hard to enter.

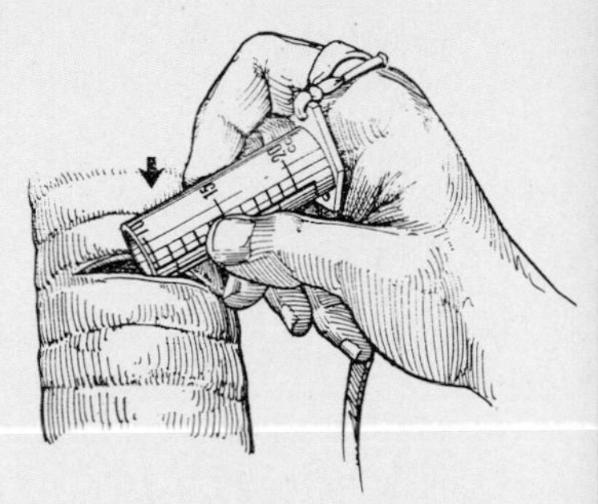

When you can feel the trachea directly, stabilize the trachea with one hand, punch into it between two tracheal rings with the point of the knife, and then enlarge the opening just enough that the syringe barrel can fit in snugly. (If you cannot get a 20 cc syringe barrel to fit without putting excessive pressure on the hard, cartilage "rings" of the trachea, use a 12 cc syringe).

Quickly check that air is moving through the syringe and pack the area between the skin edges and the syringe tightly with gauze sponges or even paper towels if nothing else is available. (Do not use cotton as it will get into the open wound and leave fibers.) The horse will arouse quickly once he gets air again.

If you cannot hear/feel air moving through the tube, check to be sure it is actually inside the trachea. If it is, pull it back slightly to make sure it is not pressed up against the wall of the trachea. If the tube fills with frothy fluid, blood or mucus, air will not be move effectively. Using a smaller syringe that will fit inside the tube, and suck out this material.

The horse must also be seen by a veterinarian as quickly as possible. Someone must stay at the horse's head at all times to make sure the tube does not come out of place before the veterinarian arrives to remove the tube and replace it with a more secure arrangement.

If the horse becomes violent, do not attempt restraint — it will be impossible. If his air becomes blocked completely and the horse collapses, you can cut into his neck and windpipe after he is unconscious to give him an airway.

All of this may sound like more than you can do. However, once the horse is down and has stopped struggling, you will be free to work. After he has regained consciousness, he will be far less likely to struggle. Someone should sit on his head to keep him down unless he is fully conscious. When he is getting up, stay close to the head at all times to keep the syringe in place until help arrives.

This procedure is definitely not something that should be attempted by anyone who is at all uneasy at the idea, as you must work quickly and surely. This is one procedure that is best discussed in advance with your veterinarian. When she is visiting, have her show you how to proceed, should you need to perform a tracheostomy.

TRAUMA TO CHEST ■■■

Open wounds/puncture wounds:

- Lung collapse is caused by wounds that penetrate through the skin and muscle of the chest wall that allow air to enter the chest cavity. Don't treat any injury that looks as if it may have penetrated into the chest. Apply pressure if the wound is bleeding. Place the horse in a quiet stall and call the vet immediately.
- Another complication may be damage to the lung tissue, which results in air escaping out of the lung. This will make its way into the chest cavity and may spread into the tissues of the wound, causing them to swell. Air in the tissues (subcutaneous emphysema) can be recognized by a characteristic crackly feel, such as with bubble wrap packing material. Emergency veterinary

attention is needed. Check with the vet about giving tetanus antitoxin and toxoid, and any antibiotic.

Blunt trauma to chest wall:

- Heavy blows or bumps to the chest wall can result in contusion of the lung, with broken ribs and/or possible bleeding into the chest cavity. The horse will show depression, reluctance to move and a very shallow breathing pattern. If the horse is in severe distress — refusing to eat or drink, with rapid and difficult breathing — emergency veterinary attention is in order.
- With less severe signs, your vet may recommend 3 grams of phenylbutazone (1,000+ pound horse) to determine how much of the symptoms are caused by pain. If the horse shows obvious relief, trauma to the muscles/bones of the chest wall is probably the major problem. If there is no significant improvement **within 24 hours**, or if the condition worsens or fever develops, call the vet.
- Talk with your vet about keeping the horse on phenylbutazone at 1 or 2 grams daily. Take his temperature before giving him each dose.

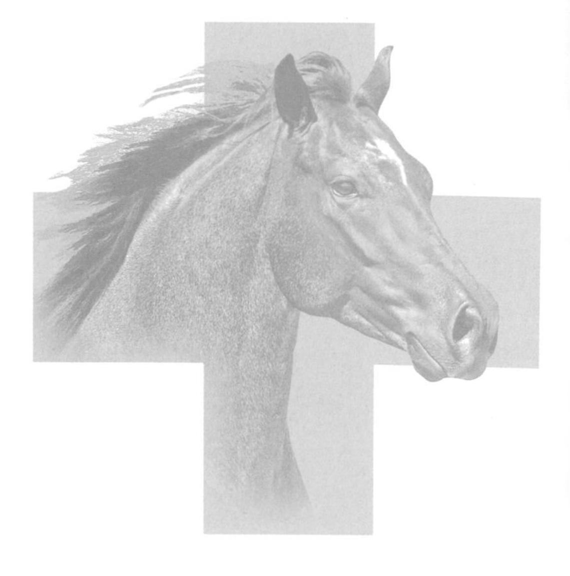

13

SEIZURES AND COLLAPSE

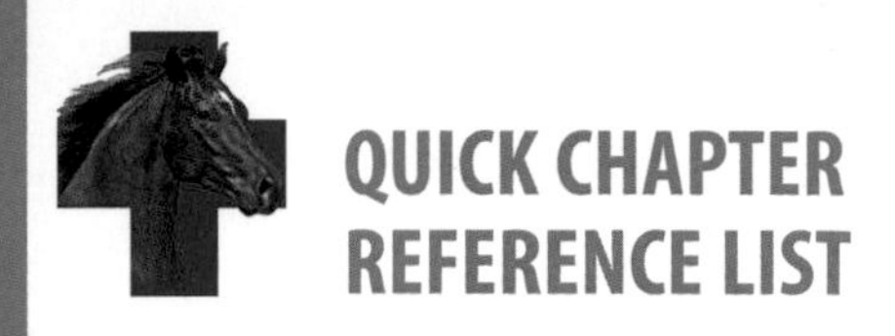

QUICK CHAPTER REFERENCE LIST

LEGEND: ■■■ — NEEDS EMERGENCY ATTENTION; ■■ — SHOULD BE EXAMINED BY A VET; ■ — MAY NEED VETERINARY ADVICE/ATTENTION

COLLAPSE

NOTE: This chapter deals with loss of consciousness and seizure activity, which occurs unexpectedly and for no apparent reason. For collapse with an obvious cause — e.g., exhaustion, heat prostration, breathing emergency — see the appropriate section.

Symptoms:

Loss of consciousness or seizure activity may occur unexpectedly or be preceded by behavior changes. It is important to note all surrounding events, before, during and after the episode, to aid in diagnosis and proper treatment. Behavior changes preceding loss of consciousness or a seizure may range from depression or blank staring to agitation and hypersensitivity to stimuli such as light, touch or sound. Loss of consciousness may last for seconds to minutes, with the horse lying quietly or showing twitching and/or thrashing movements (for seizure activity, see below). After regaining consciousness, the horse may be completely normal or may seem dazed, depressed or confused.

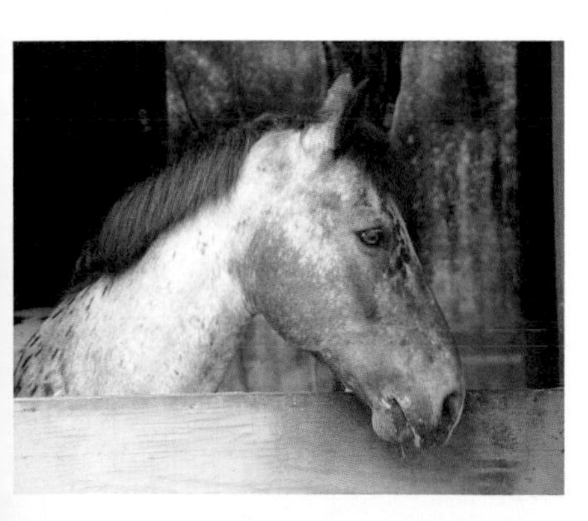

Following a seizure, the horse may be depressed and have a far-away look, or he may appear completely normal.

LOSS OF CONSCIOUSNESS ■■

Definition:
Losing consciousness or "passing out."

Possible causes:
Loss of consciousness ("fainting") could be caused by cardiac problems. It could be a type of seizure, or it could be related to a lesion in the brain following trauma. Cardiac problems or a specific disorder of the brain called narcolepsy are the most likely causes of altered consciousness without seizure movements. The horse may collapse entirely or may seem to suddenly fall asleep and buckle at the knees.

With cardiac causes, exercise may or may not precipitate the attack, depending on the nature of the specific disorder underlying the problem. With narcolepsy, there will usually be some specific stimulus that triggers the attack — eating, leading the horse, stroking the horse a particular way, etc. Older horses with pituitary tumors (Cushing's disease) sometimes develop seizures or "drop attacks."

Treatment:
No specific emergency treatment necessary. In terms of prevention, if it's possible to identify a precipitating cause, that should obviously be avoided. There is a good chance that drug therapy will be helpful, but a complete veterinary examination must first determine the cause. A detailed description of the event will aid this diagnosis.

SEIZURES/"FITS" ■■

Symptoms:
Seizure activity is an abnormal firing of nerve cells in the brain that results in loss of consciousness and any of the following signs:

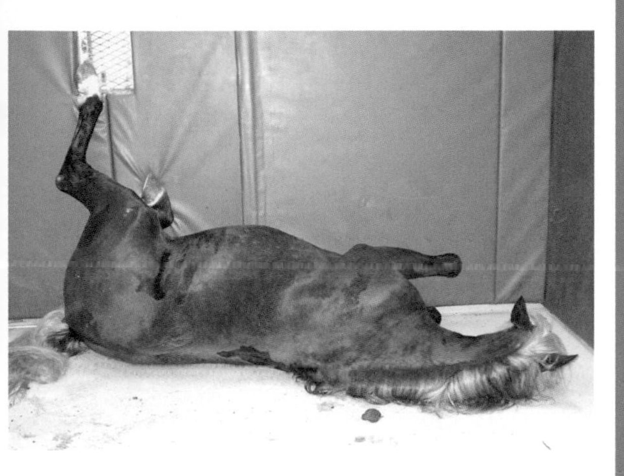

During a seizure, it is possible for the horse to injure itself or become cast in its stall.

- Twitching
- Jerking
- Collapse
- Limb movement
- Neck stiffness
- Movements of eyes and lips
- Urination
- Defecation
- Salivation
- Sweating.

Seizures may be separated by minutes, hours, days, months or even years.

Causes:

Seizures may be a congenital problem (epilepsy); secondary to damage from decreased blood supply, infection, trauma or tumor; drug reactions; related to liver failure; or may appear as the predominant symptom of rabies. Seizures may also be seen with viral encephalitis (EEE, WEE, West Nile virus).

Treatment:
No attempt should be made to restrain or "wake up" a horse having a seizure. The danger to you is too great.

After the seizure is over, remove any buckets from the stall, darken the stall and keep stimulation of any kind to an absolute minimum. Precise recording of the seizure activity is critical to diagnosis. Note particularly if the abnormal movements occurred on both sides of the body, if all parts of the body or only some were involved, or if the animal lost urine or feces during the seizure.

Because of the danger that the seizure activity could be a manifestation of rabies, extreme caution should be used because there is always a chance the horse has been exposed to a rabid animal. Do not attempt to treat any self-inflicted injury or to comfort/reassure the horse, since there is no way to predict whether another seizure is going to occur. Veterinary attention will be needed to treat the current episode, determine the cause of the seizure and institute the correct drug therapy.

Troubleshooting during recovery:
Your veterinarian may not be able to determine the cause of the seizure on the emergency visit, and will need to await the results of tests. He or she may refer you to a veterinary hospital. In the meantime, be aware that the horse could have another seizure at any time. Do not stress the horse and do not turn him out with a group. It's OK to keep any buddies nearby, though. The safest place for the horse is in a paddock with feed and water buckets hung on the outside of the fence, placed so the horse can reach over to eat and drink.

14

DISORDERS OF BALANCE, COORDINATION, PERSONALITY

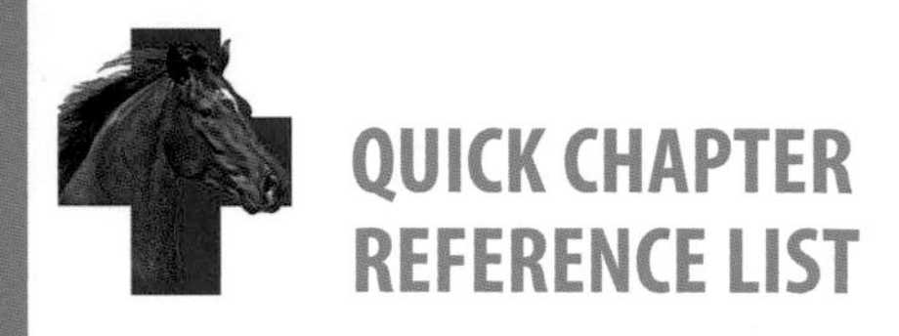

QUICK CHAPTER REFERENCE LIST

LEGEND: ■■■ — NEEDS EMERGENCY ATTENTION; ■■ — SHOULD BE EXAMINED BY A VET;
■ — MAY NEED VETERINARY ADVICE/ATTENTION

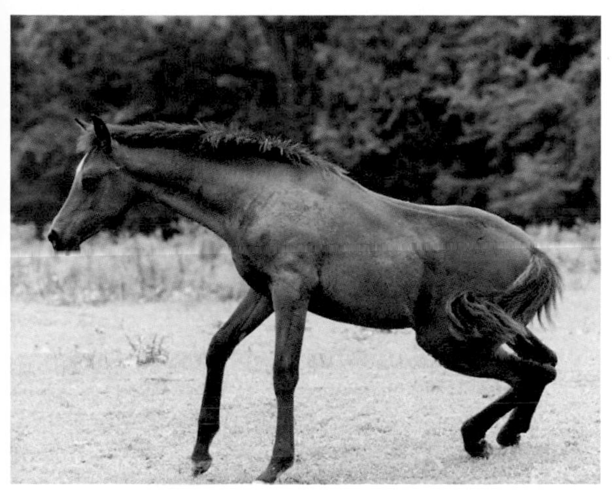

Call the vet immediately if a horse suddenly develops lack of coordination, excess salivation or hind-end weakness.

DISORDERS OF BALANCE, COORDINATION, PERSONALITY

The specialty of neurology and detail of all the possible causes for the above symptoms is too extensive to be appropriate for a first aid book. However, you should know enough about the possible causes to recognize what could produce these symptoms in your horse. Some general categories are given below.

- **Infections**: Viral, bacterial, fungal or protozoal infections can all cause central nervous system disease. The primary symptoms are usually related to loss of balance and coordination, rather than personality changes or seizures. Your vet will need to know the horse's vaccination history and any history of infectious diseases in the past, particularly respiratory infections (even if mild) or strangles.

- **Feed-related**: Moldy corn contains a toxin that destroys brain tissue. If you feed corn in any form, including a sweet feed or pellet with corn in it, this could be the source.
- **Plant poisoning**: There are several plants that can cause neurological problems. Many of these do so by causing liver damage, which allows poisons that affect the brain to build up in the body. Violent, hyperactive periods, interspersed with periods of marked depression, are the usual symptoms. The horse may injure himself badly during the violent episodes. In addition, the mucous membranes will be yellow-orange in color, and the urine will be dark.
- **Lead poisoning, tetanus, botulism** and **rabies** are all associated with varying degrees of neurological dysfunction. Loss of swallowing ability and heavy salivation are early symptoms of each disease.
- Causes within the brain itself may include tumors, injury secondary to trauma or interference with the normal blood supply.

NEUROLOGIC SYMPTOMS

Symptoms of acute neurological disease are generally very dramatic. The horse may show any of the following signs, in any combination:

- Staggering
- Standing rooted in place
- Rigid posture, reluctance to move
- Increased or decreased response to touch, sound
- Loss of coordination
- Tilting or holding head to one side
- Dragging of toes
- Circling or falling to the side
- Inability to back up
- Inability to raise the head without losing balance

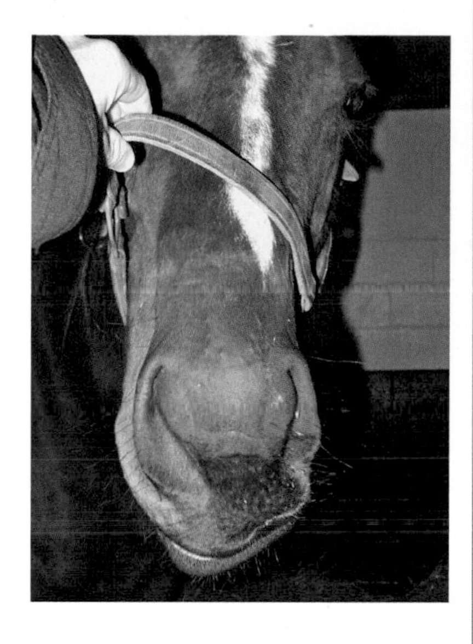

Paralysis of the horse's right facial nerve is making the muzzle look pulled to the left.

- Personality changes
  - Aggression
  - Marked depression
  - Stupor
  - Staring
  - Panic
- Apparent blindness
- Running into walls
- Pressing head against wall or the other solid object ("head pressing")
- Violent thrashing
- Twitching of face or body
- Drooping of face or ear on one side of the head
- Loss of consciousness
- Seizures.

Emergency treatment:

The onset of neurological signs is an emergency condition that calls for prompt veterinary atten-

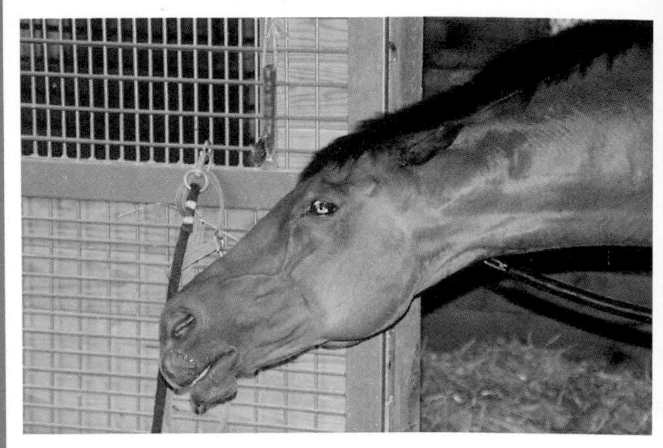

Significant personality changes may accompany neurological problems.

tion, rapid diagnosis and specific treatment if there is to be any hope of recovery.

- Put the horse in as large a stall as possible, or outside in a paddock, and remove all projections from the walls, including buckets.
- Bedding should be deep in case of falls, but not so deep that it trips the horse.
- No treatment should be given before the vet arrives.
- If rabies is a possibility, stay away from the horse.
- If signs suggesting liver disease are present, do not use any field that the horse may have been turned out in for other horses until a plant expert can check it out. If your feed contains any corn, stop using it and save a sample for analysis. It's possible for only one horse to show signs, even if all are getting the same feed.

Troubleshooting during recovery:

See Chapter 13, page 138.

- Horses that are unable to rise often develop pressure sores/rubs. Treat these with zinc oxide ointment and padding where possible.
- If the bone becomes exposed, call the vet.
- Problems with pneumonia and poor gut motility leading to colic or impaction may occur.
- Get detailed instructions on turning the horse, propping him up so that he is resting on his sternum rather than his side, and correct diet.
- If the horse shows signs of trouble breathing or abdominal pain, call the vet.

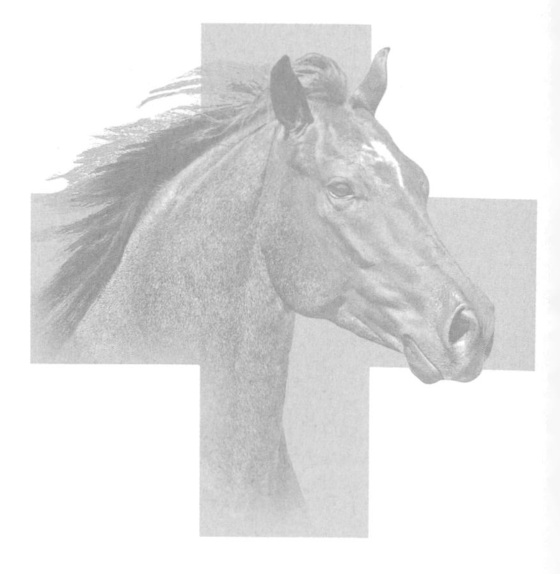

15

TRAUMA TO HEAD/NECK

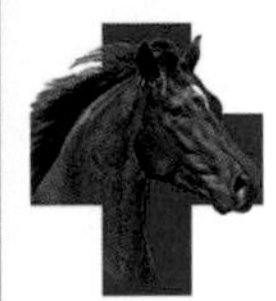

FIRST AID KIT

- Blanket
- Phenylbutazone tablets ℞
- Acepromazine tranquilizer injection ℞

℞: PRESCRIPTION DRUG — MUST BE OBTAINED FROM VETERINARIAN OR PRESCRIBED BY A VET — SHOULD NEVER BE ADMINISTERED WITHOUT PRIOR APPROVAL BY A VETERINARIAN.

QUICK CHAPTER REFERENCE LIST

LEGEND: ■■■ — NEEDS EMERGENCY ATTENTION; ■■ — SHOULD BE EXAMINED BY A VET;
■ — MAY NEED VETERINARY ADVICE/ATTENTION

TRAUMA TO THE HEAD AND NECK

BLOWS TO THE HEAD

Causes:

Blows to the head may be inflicted by humans or other horses, or they may be accidental, as when a horse rears and strikes his head or flips over backward.

Consequences:

The consequences of a severe blow to the head depend upon the area injured. Blows below the level of the eyes may injure facial bones, sinuses, or jaw. Injury to eye area may damage the eye itself (see chapter 16, page 163) or the orbit (bony socket of the eye). Blows higher on the head may injure the skull and/or brain and spinal cord.

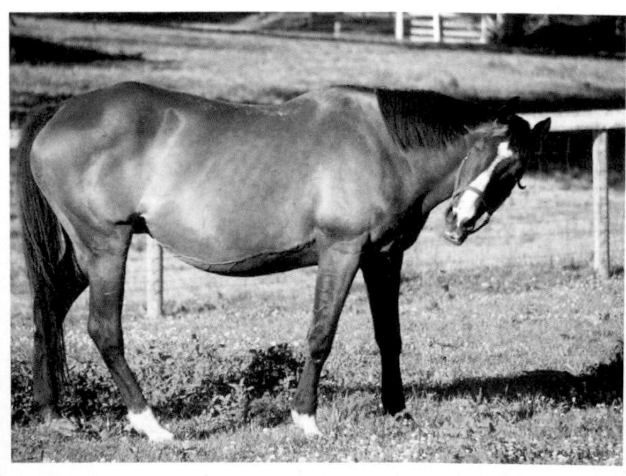

Persistently holding the head in an odd position may indicate trauma to the horse's skull or spinal cord or an inflammation of the brain.

Sinus injury/fracture ■ to ■■■

Symptoms:
Deformity of face in area of blow, bleeding from one or both nostril(s), noisy respiration, or decreased air flow from one or both nostril(s).

Complications:
Infection is likely. Pus-like drainage may begin as soon as 24 to 48 hours after the injury. Appearance of pus at the nostrils may be delayed if drainage is blocked by the injury. Observe for increased facial swelling.

Treatment:
- Nosebleed — see Chapter 5, page 50. May tranquilize horse lightly if bleeding is not profuse (get veterinary approval first).
- Remove halter if it is tight or putting direct pressure on injured area. Pad the halter well before replacing.
- Observe for signs of severe respiratory distress, i.e., depression, flared nostrils, or a respiratory rate over 25 breaths per minute at rest.
- May give one to three grams of phenylbutazone per 1,000 pounds for pain with your vet's approval.
- Monitor temperature twice daily for seven days. Prophylactic antibiotic coverage (e.g., penicillin) may be started on approval of veterinarian.

Troubleshooting during recovery:
Get veterinary attention for any of the following:
- Obvious deformity/swelling
- Noisy respiration
- Decreased air flow from one or both nostrils
- Heavy or persistent bleeding
- Temperature elevation to 101° or greater on two or more consecutive readings
- Pus or foul odor from nostrils

- Refusal to eat or drink within 12 hours of injury
- Difficulty with chewing or swallowing food/water.

Fractured jaw ■■

Symptoms:

Swelling in area of jaw, "clicking" noise on jaw movement, pain on pressure over jaw, refusal or reluctance to eat or drink.

Treatment:

Remove halter if it's putting pressure on injured area use a larger halter and pad it well before replacing. May give 1 to 3 grams of phenylbutazone per 1,000 pounds, as above, for pain. Call the vet immediately if the horse is not eating or drinking. Will need X-rays to determine treatment needed.

Troubleshooting during recovery:

Call the vet if swelling increases for no obvious reason, if the horse develops a fever or stops eating and drinking.

Injury to area of eye ■■■

Symptoms:

See Chapter 16, page 163 for injuries to the eye itself. Extreme pain, swelling or obvious deformity, bulging of eye, apparent blindness on affected side may all indicate injury to the structures around the eye.

Treatment:

Call the vet immediately if any of the above symptoms are present. Delay in treatment could result in blindness. May give 1 to 3 grams of phenylbutazone per 1,000 pounds to control pain, on vet's approval.

Troubleshooting during recovery:

Worsening of corneal edema (white eye), change in color of the cornea from white to yellow, or heavy in-growth of blood vessels into the cornea may signal uncontrolled infection. Call the vet. Also call if the size of the eye changes.

Trauma to skull/brain/spinal cord ■■■

Symptoms:

Symptoms of skull fracture include any obvious deformity of the injured area, marked swelling, or neurological signs indicating concussion or brain hemorrhage. Neurological signs include:

- Head held tilted
- Staggering, swaying
- Pupils of unequal size
- Pupils with decreased or no reaction to light
- Blood or clear fluid draining from ear.

Injuries to spinal cord high in the neck may cause the above signs plus refusal to turn or bend the neck, hold-

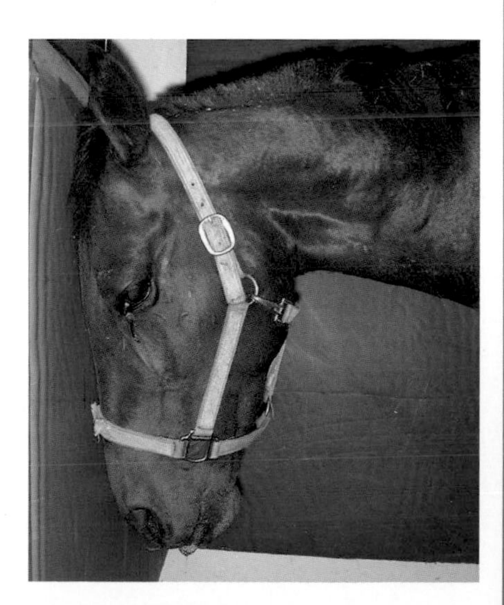

With diseases involving the brain, periods of severe depression/stupor and poor responsiveness are commonly seen, but can switch at any moment to violence and agitation.

ing the neck in a rigid position, sudden paralysis or other neurological signs (see neurological disease, page 134), or sudden death from paralysis of muscles of respiration.

Treatment:

- Do not attempt to move the horse.
- May tranquilize lightly if the horse is agitated or struggling. Try to avoid this.
- Give 2 to 3 grams of phenylbutazone per 1,000 pounds to control pain and help with inflammation.
- Blanket (according to weather) as general supportive care against shock.
- Get immediate veterinary attention.

FLIPPING OVER BACKWARD ■■■

Brain and spinal cord

Symptoms:

Injury to skull, brain, or spinal cord, as described above, is very likely.

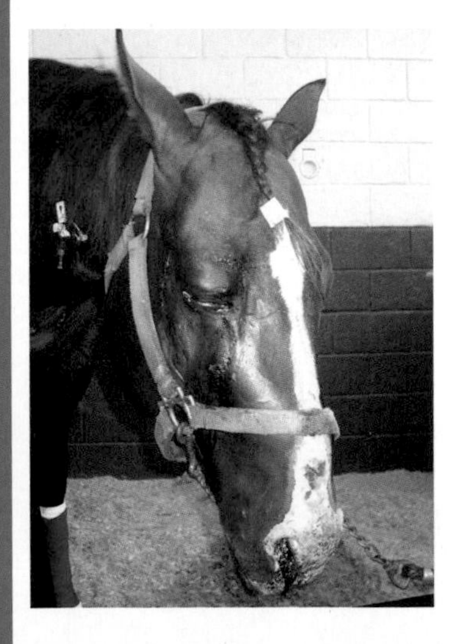

Bloody nose and facial swelling from a skull fracture.

Treatment:

Do not force horse to stand. Quietly remove any restricting equipment (side reins, etc.) and stand back. If the horse is not up in a few minutes and/or if showing any of the signs listed under trauma to skull/brain/spinal cord, treat as above.

Troubleshooting during recovery:

Swelling of the brain or spinal cord may return after the initial emergency treatment. Call the vet if symptoms start to worsen.

Other fractures

Note: Horses that go over backward may also suffer fractures of the lower spine (back and rump), pelvis, ribs, wither or other bones. Check carefully over the next few days for any areas of tenderness or swelling. Extreme muscular tenderness/spasm along the back may indicate a fracture in that area. Rapid, shallow respiration, reluctance to move, or extreme resentment of girth may indicate rib fracture. Contact the veterinarian if severe injury of this type is suspected. With your vet's approval, control pain with phenylbutazone, 1 to 3 grams once or twice daily, but no more than 4 mg/lb total daily dose.

Troubleshooting during recovery:

Call the vet if the horse's pain does not steadily improve, if new symptoms develop, or if any of the above symptoms worsen.

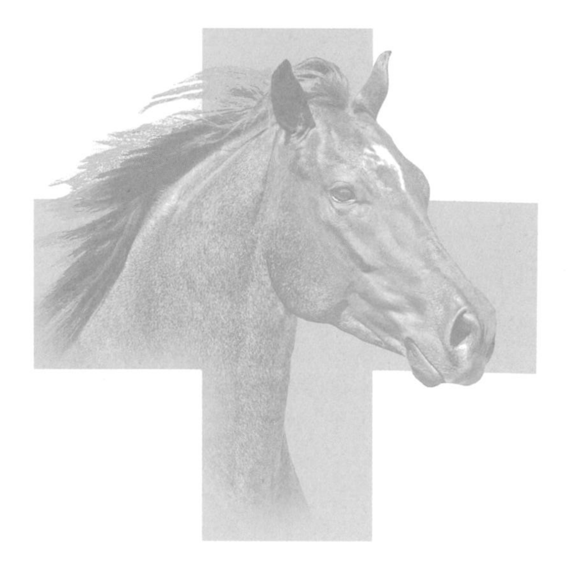

16

EYES

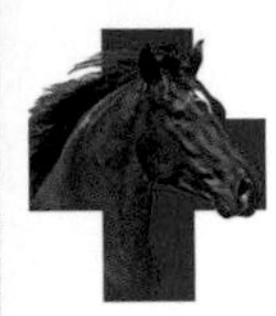

FIRST AID KIT

- Cotton swabs (Q-tips)
- Xylazine (Rompun) ℞
- Fly repellent, fly mask
- Antibiotic ophthalmic ointment or drops (no steroids added)
- Atropine ophthalmic ointment or drops ℞
- Cold compress
- Twitch

℞: PRESCRIPTION DRUG — MUST BE OBTAINED FROM VETERINARIAN OR PRESCRIBED BY A VET — SHOULD NEVER BE ADMINISTERED WITHOUT PRIOR APPROVAL BY A VETERINARIAN.

QUICK CHAPTER REFERENCE LIST

LEGEND: ■■■ — NEEDS EMERGENCY ATTENTION; ■■ — SHOULD BE EXAMINED BY A VET;
■ — MAY NEED VETERINARY ADVICE/ATTENTION

EYES

Problems that involve the eye are always emergencies. Delay in treatment can result in permanent injury to your horse's vision. If you are at all unsure what the symptoms mean, have your vet look at the eye immediately.

SWOLLEN EYE ■■ AND PROMINENT THIRD EYELID ■

Possible causes:

Insect sting, irritation from dust or insects, blow to the eye, foreign material under eyelids, or injury to eyelids or eye itself. Prominent third eyelid can also be a sign of tetanus.

Treatment:

- Restrain horse (twitch may be needed).
- Gently open eye to check for obvious damage to eye itself.
- Gently pull down lower eyelid to look for dirt, plant material or other matter. If foreign matter is identified on inner surface of eyelids, you may attempt removal by touching this gently with a dry cotton swab. Do not attempt removal of any material that is on the eye itself. Do not attempt removal if horse is not well restrained.
- Note any swelling or redness of inner surfaces of eyelids and report this to the veterinarian
- Place the horse in a dark, quiet stall. If a darkened stall is not available, tape duct tape over one side of a fly mask to provide some relief from light.

- Apply cold moist compresses to the closed eye every 15 to 20 minutes for five minutes until the veterinarian arrives. You may be able to bandage these in place, using an elastic leg wrap looped around the sides of a halter and behind the ears.

TEARING ■ TO ■■

Possible causes:
Tearing may accompany any injury to the eyelid or eye, inflammation of the eye's membranes (conjunctivitis), or may be caused by a blocked tear duct.

Treatment:
- Try to determine if the eye or eyelid is injured. If there is no obvious injury — if the horse holds his eyes wide open and he doesn't object to light — the problem is probably a blocked tear duct. The veterinarian will have to insert a small tube and flush this clear.
- If there is an injury to the eyelid or eye itself, follow instructions elsewhere in this chapter.

INABILITY TO OPEN EYELIDS ■■■

Possible causes:
Damage to facial nerve that innervates (supplies the nerves to) the muscles controlling eyelid movement causes drooping and paralysis of the eyelid. Brain tumor or infection may involve upper and/or lower eyelid.

Treatment:
- Differentiate an inability to move the lids from the horse deliberately keeping the lids shut. If the horse can't control his eyelids, you'll likely see that they're droopy and you can move them easily. If he is closing the lids deliberately, he will clamp them tighter when you try to open them.

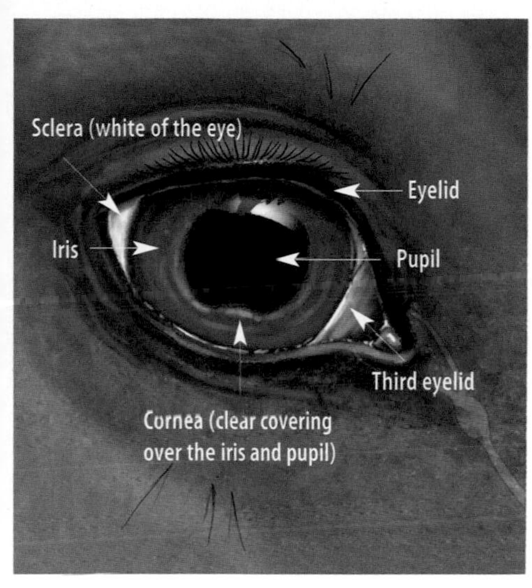

- There may also be associated paralysis of ear, nostril, or lip on the same side of the face.
- If the eye is only partially closed, it may be very dry and/or injured.
- Place the horse in a dark stall.
- Remove the halter, particularly if it's tight, as this may be placing pressure on the facial nerve.
- Contact the veterinarian.

REFUSAL TO OPEN EYELIDS ■■ TO ■■■

Possible causes:
Refusal to open eyelids indicates eye pain. This may be due to an injury to the eye or eyelids, or to a disease of the eye such as recurrent uveitis (also known as ERU, periodic ophthalmia or moon blindness).

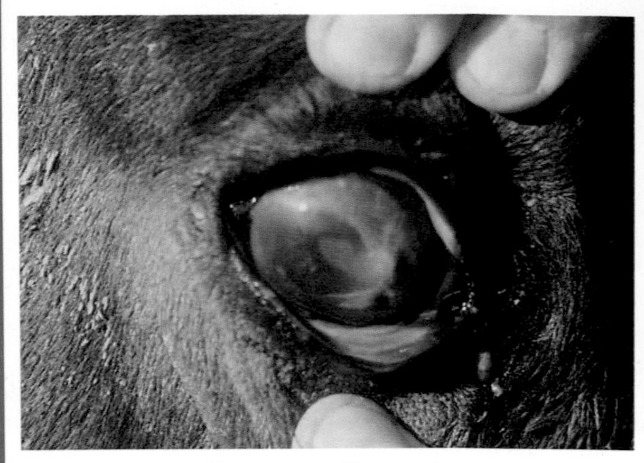

Injuries to the eye itself require immediate veterinary treatment to avoid permanent blindness.

Treatment:
Same as for swollen eye.

LACERATION TO EYELIDS ■■■

Possible causes:
Direct trauma to eye.

Treatment:
- Try to determine if the eye itself is also injured. However, do not manipulate the injured eyelid.
- Follow the same treatment as for swollen eye.

WHITE EYE OR WHITE SPOT ON EYE ■■■

Possible causes:
Whitening of the cornea occurs with direct injury to the eye or as a result of infection or inflammation, such as occurs with a systemic disease such as recurrent uveitis.

Treatment:

Same as for swollen eye. **If eye medications are available, put ophthalmic antibiotic ointment** or drops (no steroid added) into the eye every three to four hours, and atropine drops every four hours.

Troubleshooting during recovery:

Have the eye re-examined if:

- Area of whiteness increases
- Area of whiteness does not steadily decrease in size
- Whiteness changes to a grey or yellowish color
- Blood vessels start to grow into the cornea.

BLOOD IN EYE ■■■

Possible causes:

May result from trauma or as a result of problem such as periodic ophthalmia.

Treatment:

Same as for white eye.

COLLAPSED EYE ■■■

Cause:

Penetrating injury, or erosion of an ulcer on the cornea.

Treatment:

Same as for white eye. If the eye is already under treatment (as for an ulcer), call the vet for a re-evaluation for any possible changes in medications and injection of medications superficially into the sclera (white of the eye).

"BLOODSHOT" EYE

Possible causes:
Usually results from direct trauma to the eye. However, prominent blood vessels in the sclera may also be seen with other injuries or inflammations on the cornea or deep in the eye.

Treatment:
There is no specific treatment for a "bloodshot" eye. This will resolve with treatment of other concurrent problems, such as above.

PUS/WHITE MATERIAL AT CORNER OF EYE ■■

Possible causes:
Infection of any eye structures, inflammation of conjunctivae, blocked tear duct, or irritation from insects.

Treatment:
- Remove any accumulated material at frequent intervals with cool water.
- Apply fly repellents no closer than 2 inches from eyes.
- May use antibiotic ophthalmic ointment or drops every four hours.
- Call the vet to rule out a blocked tear duct and to advise on use of medications containing steroids. Equine eyes are uniquely sensitive to steroids. Severe infections may follow their use if the cornea is even slightly injured.

Troubleshooting during recovery:
Get a veterinary examination if:
- Swelling develops or increases.
- Horse starts holding the eye shut.
- Any discoloration of the cornea develops.

17

FROSTBITE AND EXPOSURE

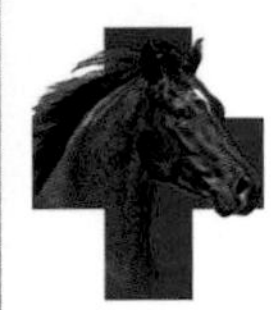

FIRST AID KIT

- Blankets
- Betadine solution
- Zinc oxide or A & D skin ointments

QUICK CHAPTER REFERENCE LIST

LEGEND: ■■■ — NEEDS EMERGENCY ATTENTION; ■■ — SHOULD BE EXAMINED BY A VET;
■ — MAY NEED VETERINARY ADVICE/ATTENTION

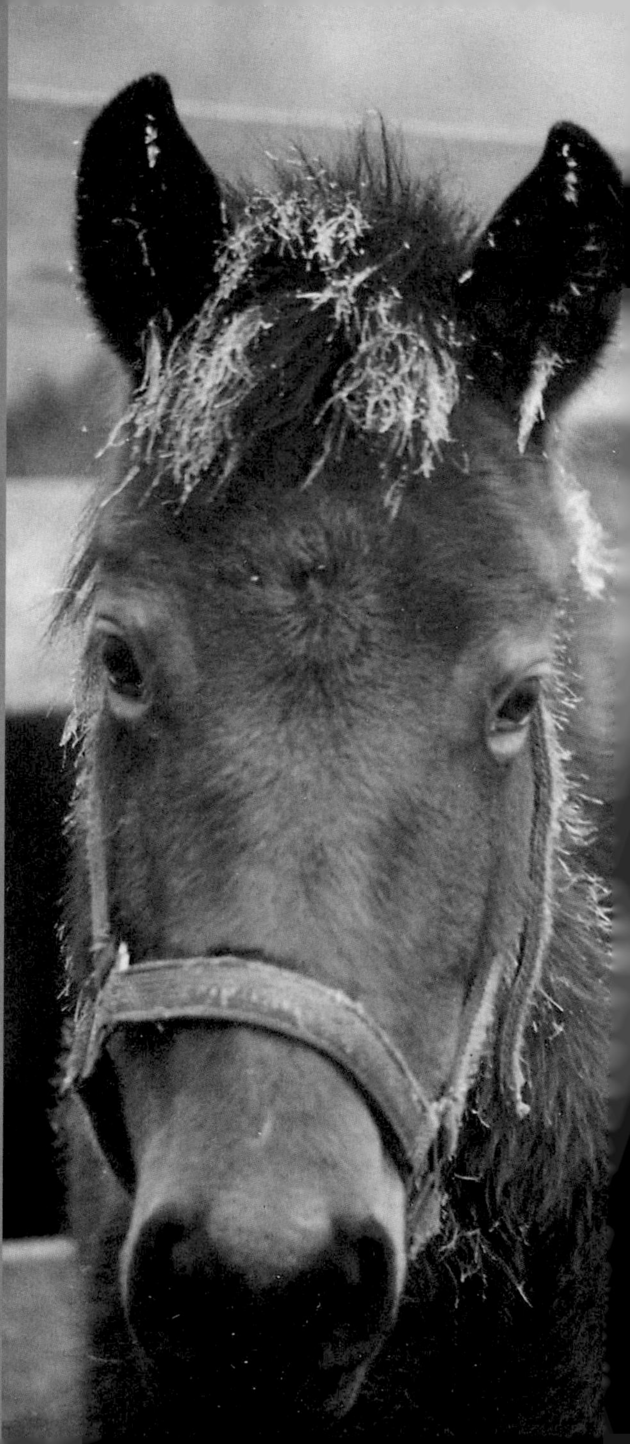

FROSTBITE AND EXPOSURE

Definition:
The destruction of superficial tissues with secondary damage to small blood vessels can result from exposure to severe cold. This is primarily a problem for foals, especially weak foals exposed to severe cold (wind chill below 0°F). Other weakened animals are also at risk.

MILD FROSTBITE ■

Signs include small crusted or scabbed areas on the muzzle, and cold ear tips with initial loss of sensation.

Treatment:
- Hold a hot pack (105 to 108° F — i.e., hot enough to feel warm on your own skin but not to burn) to affected areas for 15 to 20 minutes.
- Then apply a mild antiseptic (e.g., Betadine solution), followed by ointment such as zinc oxide or A & D.

MODERATE FROSTBITE AND EXPOSURE ■■

Signs include the above plus a depressed body temperature (below 100°F for a foal, below 98°F for an adult horse). Uncontrollable shivering may be present, with depression and sleepiness.

Treatment:
- Treat superficially damaged areas as above.
- Blanket the horse and move him to a warmed area (into a house in the case of a foal, a stall with heat

lamps and/or a nearby space heater if the animal is larger), until his body temperature is normal (minimum of 100°F for a foal, 98°F for an adult horse).

- Allow a foal free access to the mare and monitor the milk intake; call a veterinarian if the foal does not nurse in four hours.
- Offer warm water and hot mash to an adult horse.

SEVERE FROSTBITE AND EXPOSURE ■■

Signs include those for moderate frostbite and exposure, plus extremely cold feet. Feet that were kept under the body if the horse or foal was lying down will not be cold.

Treatment:

- Treat as above for moderate exposure.
- Stand the horse in buckets of warm water to encourage more rapid warming of the feet.
- If a foal is lying down, wrap warm wet packs around the feet and change frequently.
- If the horse or foal is very lethargic, call the vet for a more thorough examination and possibly warmed fluids intravenously.

Troubleshooting during recovery

Several days to weeks after the initial injury, dead tissues of the ears or feet, including hooves, may slough off.

- Sloughing off of small areas at tips of ears should be treated as any open wound.
- Animals that begin to show lameness and signs of oozing and separation at the coronary band may have to be put to sleep (euthanized). Consult with your veterinarian as to the appropriate course of action.

18

LIGHTNING AND ELECTRIC SHOCK

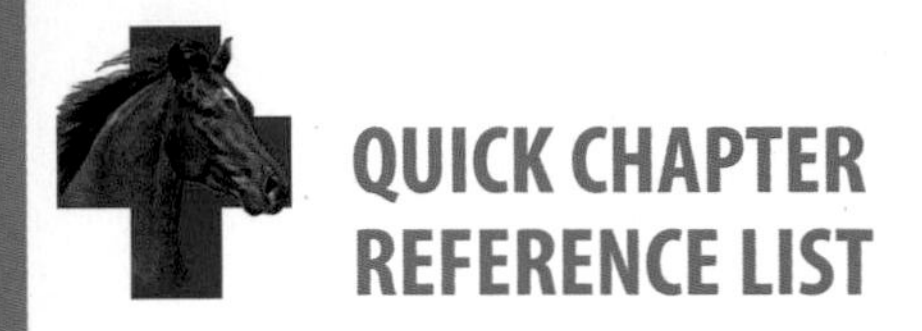

QUICK CHAPTER REFERENCE LIST

LEGEND: ■■■ — NEEDS EMERGENCY ATTENTION; ■■ — SHOULD BE EXAMINED BY A VET;
■ — MAY NEED VETERINARY ADVICE/ATTENTION

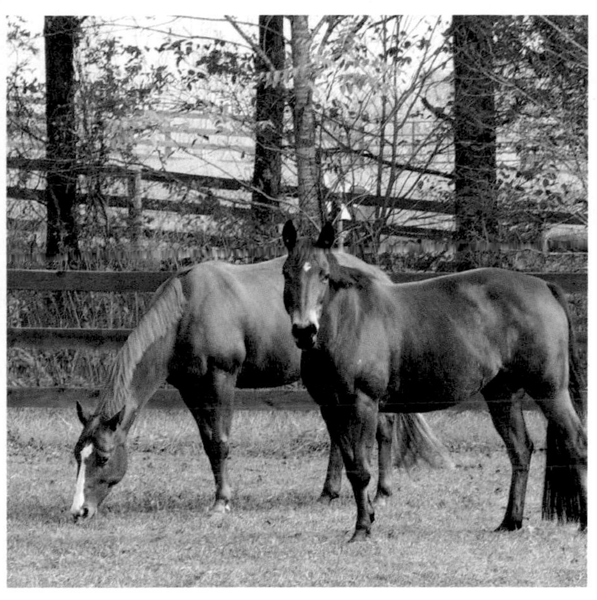

Horses caught outside during thunderstorms can be killed by lightning.

LIGHTNING AND ELECTRIC SHOCK

Injury or, more often, sudden death results from contact with high electrical current in lightning or an electrical line. Animals may be electrocuted either by direct contact with the lightning/current or by the spread of the charge. Current can travel along tree roots and may cause electrification of a shallow area of water at some distance from the actual source. Tile drains may also spread a charge. Soils vary in their conductivity, with loam being the most effective conductor, followed by clay, marble, chalk and rocky soil.

Most animals are killed if hit by lightning. A sign of electrocution is a branching, tree-like pattern of singe marks along the legs and sometimes the body. The finding of partially chewed food in the mouth and absence of any abnormal postmortem conditions also point to a sudden death, such as electrocution.

Treatment:

- Animals that do not die may be unconscious for several minutes or hours. There is no specific treatment other than general support. The animal should be kept from extremes of heat or cold, in a well-bedded stall with fresh water and high quality hay.
- Any burns should be treated as detailed in Chapter 6, page 57.

Caution: Do not touch the horse if the animal is still in contact with the electricity source.

Troubleshooting during recovery:

There may be neurological signs, such as staggering, increased sensitivity to touch or sound, and depression that persists for several days or weeks.

19

DISORDERS OF URINE/URINATION

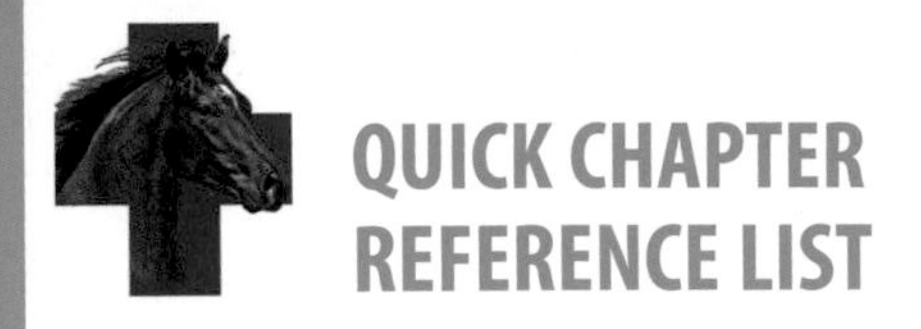

QUICK CHAPTER REFERENCE LIST

LEGEND: ■■■ — NEEDS EMERGENCY ATTENTION; ■■ — SHOULD BE EXAMINED BY A VET; ■ — MAY NEED VETERINARY ADVICE/ATTENTION

DISORDERS OF URINE/URINATION

STRAINING TO URINATE ■ to ■■

Signs:
Frequent stretching out as if to urinate (e.g., extending hind legs and dropping of the penis or opening of the lips of vulva) without passage of urine or with only a few drops of urine.

Causes:
- Nonspecific abdominal pain
- Estrus (heat) in mares
- Tying up
- Laminitis
- Bladder infection

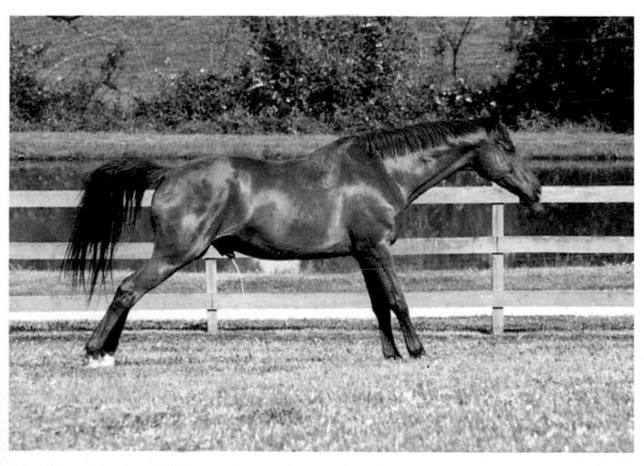

Shortly after stretching out to urinate, the horse should release urine in a constant, forceful stream.

- Stones in bladder or urethra (tube leading to outside from bladder)

Treatment:

- Try to rule out colic (see Chapter 7, page 73), tying up (only an issue if the horse has just exercised — see Chapter 11, page 118), laminitis (see Chapter 9, page 100), and estrus behavior.
- Check the stall to see if it is as wet as normal, i.e., if the horse has been urinating.
- Observe the horse carefully to see if he's able to urinate. If a blockage is suspected, get immediate veterinary attention. Urinary blockages are extremely rare in mares, but more likely in geldings.
- Do not use home remedies or over-the-counter remedies for "kidney problems." These do not work and will cause delay in treatment of a possible blockage.
- If the horse is urinating, try to catch a sample for analysis. (Moving the horse to a stall with clean bedding often triggers urination.)

Troubleshooting during recovery:
If a blockage is found and relieved, the horse should be watched closely for the next 24 hours. If your vet has inserted a catheter, there may be swelling of the tissues caused by its passing. That swelling can itself obstruct flow, and any remaining thick sediment in the bladder may cause another blockage.

FREQUENT URINATION ■ to ■■

Signs: Same as above, with passage of small amount of urine each time.
Causes: Same as above.
Treatment: Same as above.

DISCOLORED URINE

■ to ■■

Definition:
Passage of urine that is any color other than yellow or whitish.

Causes:

Normal horse urine is yellow to whitish, the white color being due to the large amount of crystals normally present. Urine may be very dark if it is highly concentrated, such as the first urine of the morning or if water intake has not been adequate. Dark urine may also occur with destruction of red blood cells (red cell pigment), liver disease (bile pigment), or muscle breakdown (muscle pigment). Red urine may also be seen with bladder infections or stones, or with tumors of the urinary tract (which are rare).

Treatment:

- Take the horse's temperature (it may be elevated if he has an infection).
- Observe for signs of colic from urinary tract pain.
- If you can, obtain a sample of urine for the veterinarian to analyze. (Bring this to the vet's office. That may save a farm call and allow the vet to prepare for any necessary further work-up).

Troubleshooting during recovery:
If a urinary tract infection is found and treated, improvement in symptoms should be obvious within 24 to 48 hours. If not, let the vet know. Also observe for symptoms returning in the first few days after you complete antibiotics.

"SORE KIDNEYS"

Definition:
"Sore kidneys" is a term horsemen often use to refer to tenderness along the topline of the back, in the general area of the saddle.

Causes:

Tenderness in this area is caused by back strain, either from pulling a load, lameness in the hind legs causing the horse to move stiffly and abnormally, or primary back muscle stiffness due to underlying spinal problems. It is rarely a sign of kidney problems. If any other signs of urinary problems are present, obtain a urine sample for analysis.

Troubleshooting during recovery:
For muscular pain, rest the horse for three days, massage his back with strong liniment after applying moist hot towels three times a day. Discontinue the liniment if the horse begins to show signs of pain when you apply it (tail swishing, kicking, moving away) but continue with the hot towels three times a day. Keep the horse blanketed in cool weather, and with your vet's approval give him phenylbutazone, 2 grams once daily (1,000+ pound horse). If there is no improvement after three days, get a veterinary evaluation. Have the horse's saddle checked for correct fit.

20
REPRODUCTIVE ORGANS

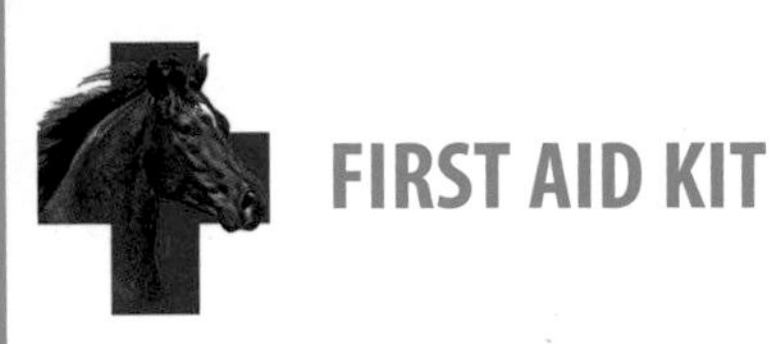

FIRST AID KIT

- Flunixin meglumine (Banamine) ℞
- Phenylbutazone ℞
- Antibiotic ointment
- Sling for penis

℞: PRESCRIPTION DRUG — MUST BE OBTAINED FROM VETERINARIAN OR PRESCRIBED BY A VET — SHOULD NEVER BE ADMINISTERED WITHOUT PRIOR APPROVAL BY A VETERINARIAN.

QUICK CHAPTER REFERENCE LIST

LEGEND: ■■■ — NEEDS EMERGENCY ATTENTION; ■■ — SHOULD BE EXAMINED BY A VET;
■ — MAY NEED VETERINARY ADVICE/ATTENTION

REPRODUCTIVE ORGANS

DROPPED PENIS ■■

Definition:
The correct term for a persistently dropped penis is paraphimosis (often a temporary condition) or priapism (a paralyzed penis).

Causes of Paraphimosis:

Trauma or infection of penis/sheath, or drug reaction (phenothiazine tranquilizers), Equine Infectious Anemia (EIA), purpura hemorrhagica (reaction to a strep infection), rhinopneumonitis, exhaustion, starvation, or paralyzed penis.

Treatment of paraphimosis:

- With trauma or infection of the penis or sheath, the area should be cleaned well and hosed with cold water for 15 to 20 minutes four times daily to minimize edema.
- With infection or direct injury to the penis, the penis should be coated with an antibiotic ointment and antibiotic injections may be indicated. Anti-inflammatory therapy with phenylbutazone or Flunixin meglumine is indicated for three to five days. Check with your vet about dosages.
- Supporting the penis in a sling — either a specifically manufactured stallion support or a sheet tied around the belly — may be needed. Get a veterinary examination.
- With paraphimosis of other causes, support and time are the only treatments.

Causes of Priapism:

Injury to local nerves, rabies, phenothiazine tranquilizers.

Treatment of Priapism:

True penile paralysis is treated by amputation of the penis, after the stage of acute inflammation caused by blood pooling has subsided. In the interim, support of the penis is indicated.

TRAUMA TO PENIS ■■

See paraphimosis, above.

SWELLING OF SHEATH (PREPUCE) ■

Causes:

- May be caused by injury or by a collection of secretions in the sheath and secondary skin irritation and infection. The surface of the extended penis will be covered with flaky and/or tarry material.

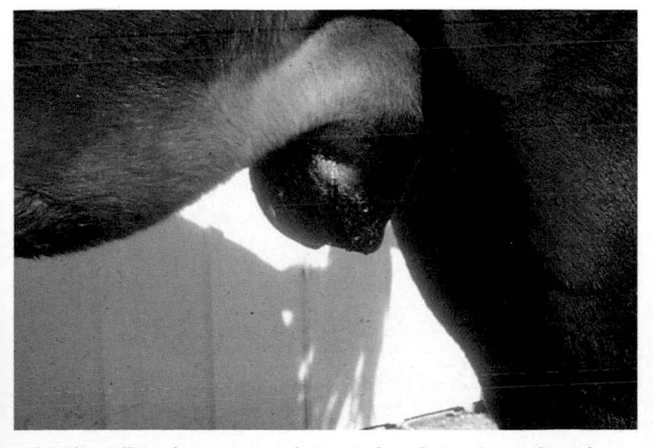

A sheath swelling that prevents the penis from being dropped needs immediate attention.

- Allergic reactions to fly bites are a fairly common cause of sheath swelling in the summer.
- Sheath swelling may also occur because of heavy deposits of fat in this area.
- If the sheath is found to be clean and free of any injuries, the horse should be tested for Cushing's disease and insulin resistance.

Treatment:

With trauma or infection of the penis or sheath, the area should be cleaned well with a sheath-cleaning product or very gentle soap (such as Ivory) and hosed with cold water. Hose the sheath area with cold water for 15 to 20 minutes four times daily to minimize edema.

TRAUMA TO VULVA ■■

Causes:

Trauma to the vulva can occur during breeding, foaling (see Chapter 21, page 177), abuse by caretakers, or accidental injury.

Treatment:

- Clean area with gentle soap and hose with cold water three times daily for 15 to 20 minutes.
- Extensive tears will require suturing.
- Superficial lacerations should be covered with an antibiotic ointment.

Troubleshooting during recovery:

After 24 to 48 hours, call the vet if the swelling does not improve, if a discharge develops, or if existing discharge fails to improve.

COLIC FOLLOWING BREEDING ■■■

Cause: Perforation of vagina by penis.

Treatment:

Any colic occurring within 24 hours of breeding is a medical emergency. It could be from perforation of the vagina. The penis carries contamination directly into the abdominal cavity, and an extensive, life-threatening infection results. Do not attempt to treat this on your own.

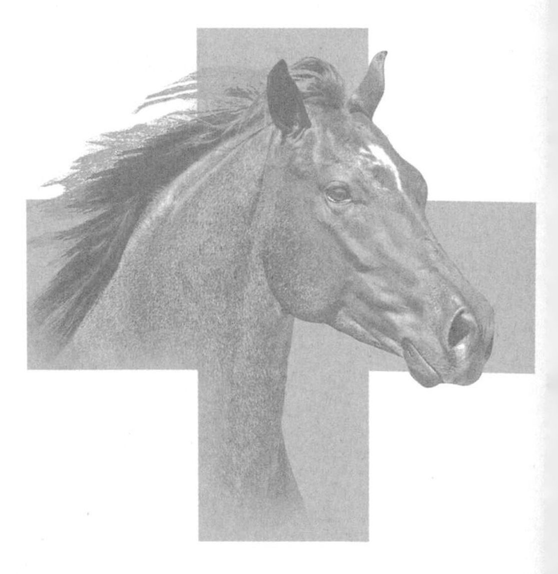

21
FOALING

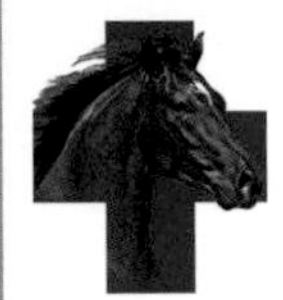

FIRST AID KIT

- Large amount of sterile lubricant, such as K-Y Jelly
- Several heavy towels
- Blanket
- Acepromazine or xylazine tranquilizer ℞
- Banamine for pain relief ℞
- Rubber gloves with textured fingers
- Sterile knife

℞: PRESCRIPTION DRUG — MUST BE OBTAINED FROM VETERINARIAN OR PRESCRIBED BY A VET — SHOULD NEVER BE ADMINISTERED WITHOUT PRIOR APPROVAL BY A VETERINARIAN.

QUICK CHAPTER REFERENCE LIST

LEGEND: ■■■ — NEEDS EMERGENCY ATTENTION; ■■ — SHOULD BE EXAMINED BY A VET;
■ — MAY NEED VETERINARY ADVICE/ATTENTION

FOALING

PROLONGED LABOR/ FAILURE OF FOAL TO APPEAR ■■ to ■■■

Definition:
Active labor with straining for longer than 20 to 25 minutes, with no placenta or parts of the foal visible.

Treatment:

- Allow the mare to roll if she wants to. This is a natural response and helps to reposition a foal that is not properly aligned in the birth canal.
- Check the vagina to make sure it has not been partially sewn shut (Caslick's operation is a common procedure to help prevent infections). If she is sewn up, you will have to open this along the scar by inserting one clean hand in the vagina and spreading the fingers just behind the vaginal opening to stretch the tissues tight. The center of the sutured area will be evident as a thin, white scar. The scar has no sensation and can be cut with scissors.
- Wrap the mare's tail and wash the genital area with mild soap, then rinse with water. Wash your hands and arms and apply K-Y Jelly, clean Vaseline or other lubricant (an appropriate lubricant should always be part of your foaling kit).
- Insert a hand in the vagina and feel around for the foal's feet or nose or any part of the foal. Foals are seldom too large to fit through the birth canal, as long as they are positioned properly.
- If you can feel part of the foal in the vagina, push it back into the uterus as far as possible during a rest period between the mare's contractions and straining.

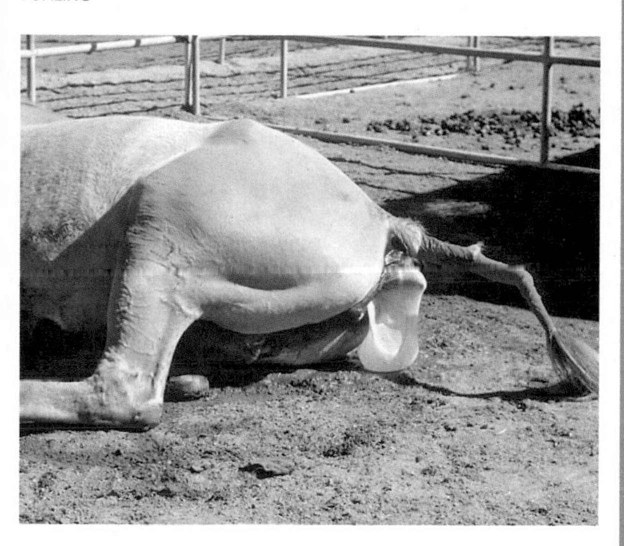

In a normal delivery, the first thing you will see is the clear amniotic sac and one or both front feet.

Then allow the mare to move around and roll. Never push the foal around or force your hand/arm through a tight area during a contraction.

When to call the veterinarian:
With this, or any problem with foaling, call the vet as soon as you suspect a problem. It is also a good idea to locate any local horseman or other livestock owners experienced in foaling or calving who might be available to help on short notice.

IMPROPER POSITION OF FOAL ■■ to ■■■

Most foals are born with their nose resting on the front legs and one foot slightly further forward than the other. However, they can also be born hind legs first without a problem. When the feet first appear, it may look as if the foal is lying on his side, or even upside down. However, this too will correct itself as the foal moves further along.

If only one foot is present, the other leg may be hung up at the elbow or hock. To correct this, the foal must be pushed back into the uterus, as described above, and the trapped leg then grasped above the foot and pulled forward. This is best done grasping the foot above the trapped fetlock and pulling out and down toward the mare's hocks. Again, intervention by experienced personnel is preferred, but you cannot afford to wait too long if the foal is already partially along the birth canal, as the umbilical cord is being compressed.

FAILURE OF FOAL TO ADVANCE ■■ to ■■■

- Occasionally, part of the foal will be visible but delivery becomes arrested. If both legs are in the birth canal, allow the mare to attempt to deliver the foal. If the foal is still not advancing, you will need to help her by pulling (with contractions) as below.
- The foal's hocks or elbows will sometimes hang up temporarily at the edge of the pelvic bone. Occasionally, the foal will become trapped at the shoulders. If this happens, the foal will have the neck and most of the front legs out. To correct this, push the foal back into the uterus several inches, then grasp one foot and pull it until the legs are positioned with one foot about six inches in front of the other. This will allow one shoulder at a time to enter the pelvis. Once the foal is positioned, grasp the legs and gently pull down toward the hocks as the mare strains to deliver the foal. Follow the same procedure if the foal is presenting hind legs first and is hung up at the pelvis.
- If only one foot can be seen and felt, the other one needs to be located and brought forward.

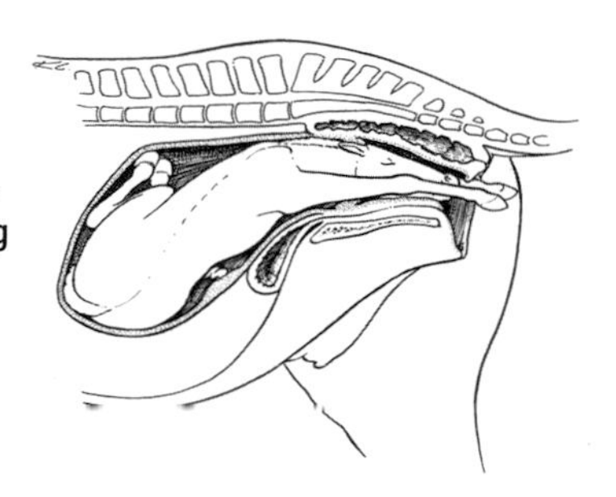

A foal in normal position, with feet in vagina during labor.

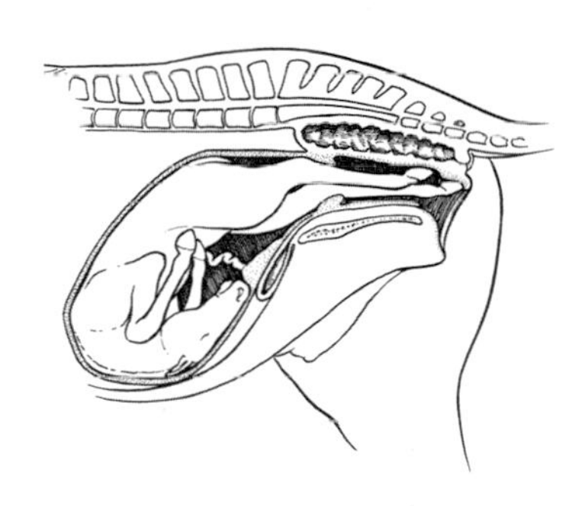

A hind feet first presentation of a foal.

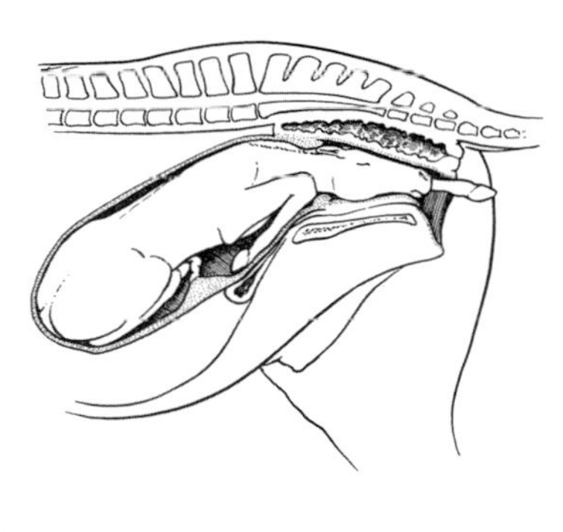

A foal, with one front leg in a normal presentation and the other flexed back under the body. His chest/shoulder area pressed against the brim of the pelvis, and the other foot normally positioned in birth canal.

Treatment:

- Push the foal back into the uterus, as far as possible between contractions.
- Follow the leg that you can already see up to the body.
- Keeping your hand on the foal's chest (or hindquarters), feel along to the other side and locate the other leg.
- Follow this leg down to the foot.
- Cup the foot in the palm of your hand and rotate it away from the foal's body and toward the flank of the mare while pushing back on the body with the other hand.
- Carefully pull the foot and leg toward you until the leg is straight.
- Delivery can then proceed normally.

The above described maneuver is difficult to perform and will seem to take forever. However, if you remain calm and proceed slowly and cautiously, the chance of success is good. If you are unable to accomplish this, or don't feel comfortable trying, keep pushing the foal back into the uterus as far as possible until help arrives. Remember, never push against a mare's contractions. Never use extreme force for any maneuvers.

UTERINE EXHAUSTION ■■

With prolonged and difficult labors, the uterus may cease to contract and the mare may lose the urge to push. If the foal is not positioned correctly, this condition actually benefits the person trying to manipulate the foal, as there will be no resistance. Regardless of how the foal is positioned, it will have to be delivered by the birth attendant.

Treatment:

- Grasp the foal's two front legs at the pastern or above the fetlocks, keeping one leg slightly behind the other,

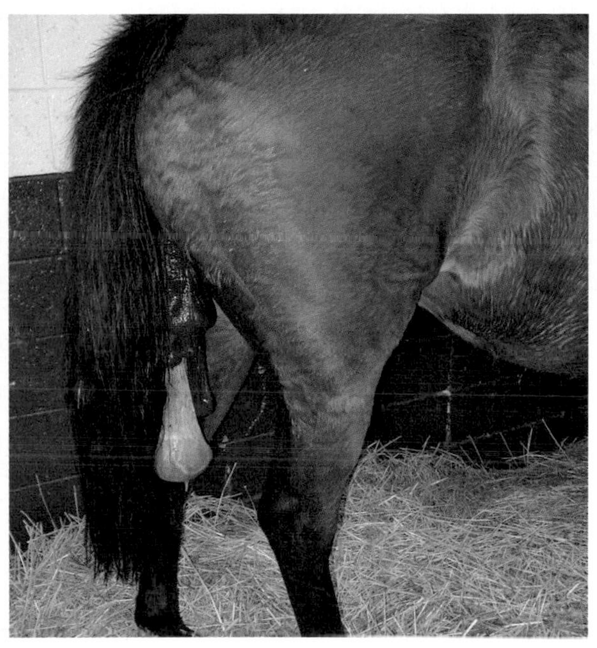

If the mare fails to pass the placenta after foaling, never pull on it

and exert a gentle, steady pull down on an angle parallel with the hocks. If the foal is too slippery, try a pair of rubber kitchen/utility gloves with textured fingers to get a better grip, or wrap small, clean hand towels around the foal's legs.

- If the mare is standing (and they often are with a hard labor), someone should be positioned to break the foal's fall and prevent sudden rupture of the umbilical cord.
- Do not cut the cord; allow it to break naturally in the course of the foal moving around. Then tie it off (if bleeding) about two inches from the foal's belly with heavy cord or baling twine. **Do not** pull on the placenta to remove it. This can cause it to break.

PREMATURE RUPTURE OF CORD ■■

Normally, the umbilical cord will break on its own as the mare and foal move around. Never cut the umbilical cord. Always let it break free on its own. Blood continues to exit the placenta and enter the foal after birth for 10 minutes or so. If it ruptures too early, heavy bleeding could occur, and blood that should have gone into the foal will be lost. The foal may then be weak, short of breath, and have difficulty standing and nursing (see below). If the foal has not made substantial efforts to stand in two hours and nurse within three hours, get emergency veterinary attention.

FAILURE OF MEMBRANES TO RUPTURE ■■

On rare occasions, the foal may be born without rupture of the inner membrane of the placenta. This is a thin, translucent sac covering the foal. If the sac remains over the foal's head, he will not be able to breathe.

What to do:

- You do not have to break the sac during the delivery process.
- If the foal has been delivered but the sac is still covering his nostrils, pull it up away from the foal and open it with your fingers, making sure it is clear of the nostrils.

RED BAG DELIVERY (PLACENTA PREVIA) ■■■

Another rare complication is red bag delivery. Instead of seeing the thin, whitish membranes containing the foal, when the mare strains, you will see a deep red, velvety tissue. This is the outer layer of the placenta that normally is ruptured when labor starts, allowing the foal and the thin sac to pass through, while the outer placenta remains firmly attached to the lining of the uterus. When this part of the placenta separates prematurely, the foal's supply of oxygen is then partially or completely cut off. In some cases, the foal is already dead. If still alive, the foal must be delivered immediately.

What to do:

- This layer of the placenta is thick and cannot be opened by hand. Pinch off a several-inches-long segment, making sure the foal is not lying directly under it, and open it with a knife or any other object you can find to penetrate it (e.g., screwdriver, hoof pick).
- Reach inside to feel for the amnionic sac, the thin membrane around the foal. Open that by hand.
- Check to see if the foal is in the correct position for delivery (see page 201). If not, correct the position.
- Immediately deliver the foal.
- If the foal is still alive, make sure the nostrils are well cleared of fluid and any memberane. Gently stimulate the foal by rubbing briskly with a towel.

Troubleshooting after delivery:

- Red bag deliveries are definitely emergencies. You still need the vet even if you have delivered the foal.
- Foals of red bag deliveries may need care in an

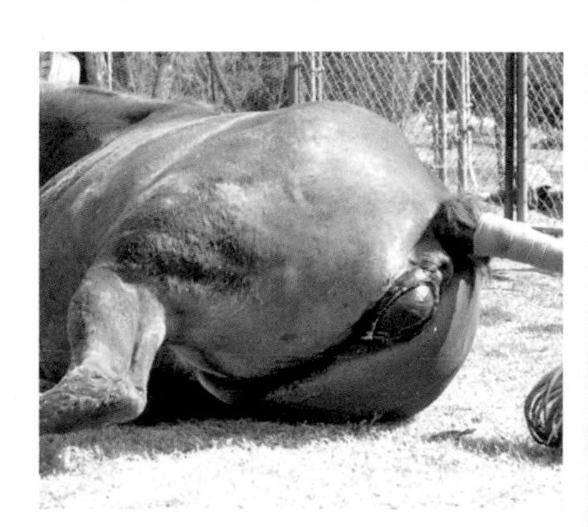

Red bag delivery. Call the vet immediately.

intensive care nursery setting. The foal needs veterinary examination to determine its status.

- Mares may lose considerable blood from uterine hemorrhage. The mare also needs to be examined by a vet.

WEAK MARE POSTPARTUM ■■■

The mare is normally quite tired after foaling and will remain lying down for around 20 minutes or so. This is beneficial, as it allows all the blood from the placenta time to enter the foal before movement of dam and foal causes the cord to break. However, if the mare stays down longer than 30 minutes, there's a possibility of internal injuries or hemorrhage.

Treatment:

- Take the mare's pulse, temperature, and respiration. These should be in the normal range in about 20 minutes after foaling.
- Check the color of the mucous membranes of her mouth. If they are very pale, suspect hemorrhage.
- Observe the mare's general attitude. Even if still down, she should be alert and looking back at the foal, calling the foal or nuzzling it.
- If she is depressed, anxious, or oblivious to the foal, this is abnormal. Relay the above information to the veterinarian.
- Dry the foal with a thick towel if the mare has not dried the foal. Place the foal close to her body, preferably where it can nurse when lying down. Remain with the mare and foal, ready to move the foal to a safe spot if the mare struggles, kicks, rolls or attempts to get up.
- Blanket the mare.

RETAINED PLACENTA ■■

The see-through, whitish membrane covering the foal when he is born is only part of the placenta. The portion that was actually attached to the uterus is still inside the mare. The mare will pass the rest of the placenta ("afterbirth") either while she is still lying down after delivery or soon after she gets up. If she does not, serious infection can set in quickly and there is a high risk of laminitis.

Treatment:

- After the mare is standing, if the placenta remains inside her, tie a knot in the umbilical cord and any visible membranes to prevent the mare from stepping on them but do **not** pull on the placenta to try to remove it. This can cause it to tear. If the mare has not passed the membranes within 2 hours of foaling, call your vet.
- When the placenta is passed, it should always be checked carefully to make sure it is all there. Spread the placenta out and you will see that it is "Y" shaped. One side will be longer and wider than the other. This is the side where the foal's body was positioned. The part of the "Y" where the umbilical cord is found is the body. The other arms of the "Y" are from the two uter-

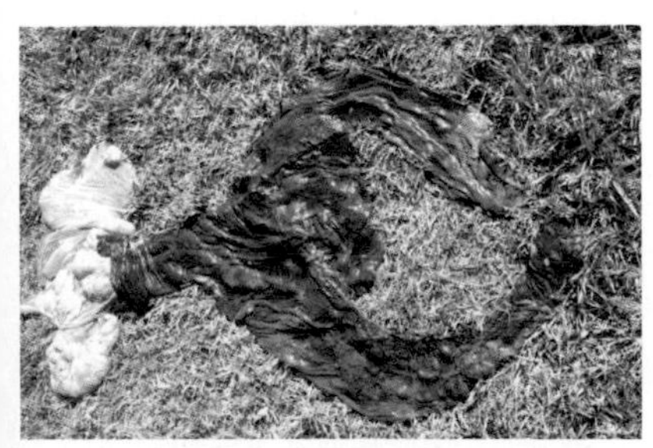

The whitish, transparent portion is the amnionic sac, the layer directly covering the foal. The red portion is the chorion, the placental membranes attached to the inside of the mare's uterus. After the mare passes her placenta, you should spread it out on the ground as shown here to make sure there are no pieces missing. If in doubt, save it for the vet.

ine horns. You will find a hole where the foal broke through but otherwise there should be no tears or missing pieces. If unsure that the placenta is all there, save it for your vet.

COLIC IN MARE POSTPARTUM ■■■

Signs of colic in the mare may be due to contractions of the uterus, possible injury to abdominal organs or hemorrhage. (See page 206 for what to do if the mare is down.) If the mare is up and agitated, care must be taken that she does not injure the foal. With your vet's approval, banamine (0.5 mg/lb) may be tried to control any pain, but tranquilizers should be avoided. If the mare becomes too violent, remove the foal to outside the stall door, but leave the door open. Have someone hold the foal and another person remain at the doorway to control the mare, if necessary. This arrangement protects the foal but limits separation anxiety.

REJECTION OF FOAL ■■

Some mares will reject their foals. This is more common with maiden mares, but may happen at any time, with any mare. The mare may refuse to have anything to do with the foal or may only resist having it nurse. Try having someone hold up one of the mare's front legs while you milk out some colostrum and then allow the foal to nurse when she has accepted this. If she's still actively resistant, a low dose of tranquilizer may be needed to overcome anxiety and allow the mare and foal to bond. If this is given within two to three hours of birth, the udder will still be full and minimal amounts of tranquilizer will reach the foal. Use 10 to 20 mg. of Acepromazine or 100 mg. of xylazine intramuscularly, per your vet's approval.

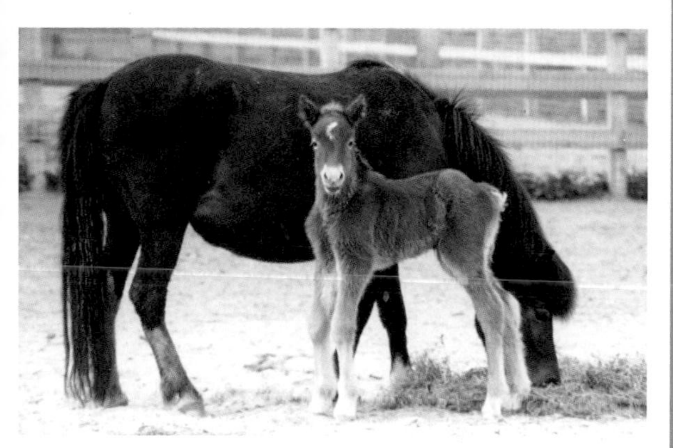

Sometimes a maiden mare needs a little help learning to accept her foal.

After the tranquilizer has taken effect, someone should stand at the mare's head while another person helps the foal to nurse. If this barrier can be overcome, the mare will sometimes grant a grudging acceptance of the foal that at least is sufficient for the foal to survive. If she is still actively resistant, seek professional advice immediately.

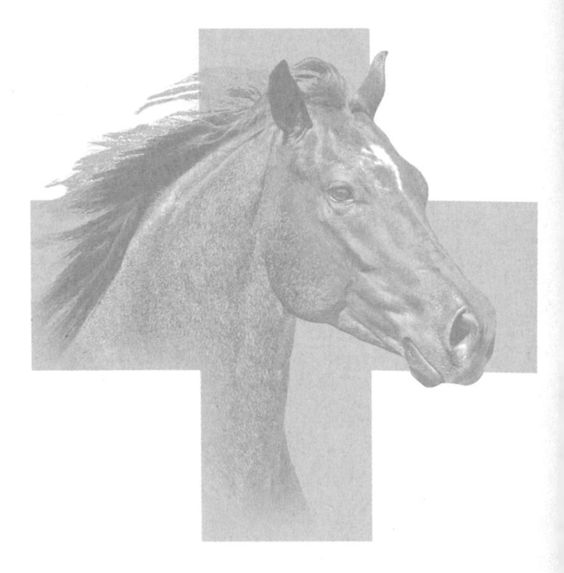

22
NEWBORN EMERGENCIES

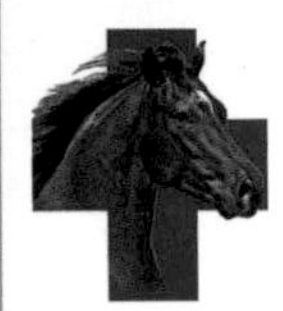

FIRST AID KIT

- Enemas
- Glycerin suppositories
- Thermometer
- K-Y jelly or Vaseline
- Human enema kit (e.g., Fleet's)
- Heat lamp

QUICK CHAPTER REFERENCE LIST

LEGEND: ■■■ — NEEDS EMERGENCY ATTENTION; ■■ — SHOULD BE EXAMINED BY A VET; ■ — MAY NEED VETERINARY ADVICE/ATTENTION

NEWBORN EMERGENCIES

The normal newborn foal is lively, alert, and very active. Although his initial attempts to stand are wobbly and uncoordinated, he makes repeated and energetic tries. The first 6 to 12 hours after birth are critical. The foal must receive the mare's first milk (colostrum) well within this time frame, and in adequate amounts to obtain the rich supply of antibodies it contains. The foal's energy, electrolyte, and fluid levels are also low, and intake of the mare's milk is essential to life. If you suspect the foal is not normal, it's best to get immediate veterinary attention so that steps can be taken to get the first milk into the foal and to evaluate him to try to uncover and correct the problem.

FAILURE TO STAND ■■■

The foal's first attempt to stand usually occurs within 30 to 60 minutes after birth. He may begin by hopping around like a gigantic frog, but eventually he gets several legs, then all four, under him. His stance at first is wide-based (splayed out) but comes to resemble normal as the foal gains strength and confidence.

When to get help:

- The time from birth to standing is highly variable. However, if the foal appears normal but hasn't managed to stand in two hours, you can assist him to his feet and help to steady him. Once this barrier is passed, a normal foal will quickly become more proficient and able to accomplish this on his own.
- If the foal is weak, disinterested, or seems depressed, place several of your fingers in his

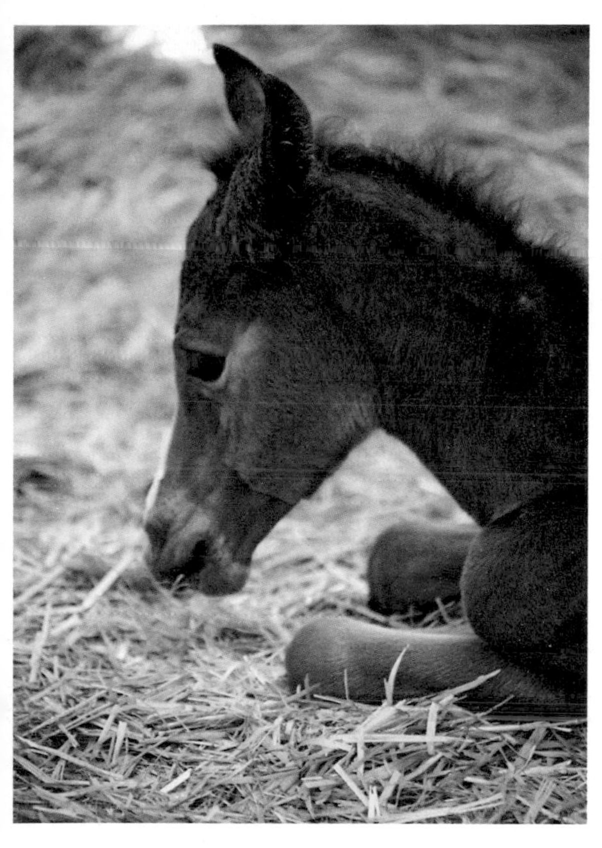

Call for veterinary help if the foal is depressed and weak 20 to 30 minutes after birth.

mouth. If he has a good, strong sucking reflex, he may be able to nurse if you hold him up to the mare's udder. Once he has nursed (note for how long and at what age, in hours, this occurred), seek veterinary attention if he is not significantly stronger after 20 to 30 minutes.

- If the foal wasn't able to nurse well, you will need veterinary assistance to pass a stomach tube to feed him.

FAILURE TO NURSE ■■■

If the foal has successfully gained his feet but has not nursed or attempted to nurse in two hours, guide him back to the udder and express a little milk onto your fingers. Once the foal is sucking your fingers, bring them close to the udder. Slide your fingers out of the way and gently guide the nipple into his mouth. (This sounds easier than it is — be patient.) Once a normal foal has successfully nursed, he is unlikely to have further problems.

If the foal is up and moving but seems abnormal in any way — wandering around, bumping into things, making abnormal sounds — and cannot be guided to nurse, as described above, get immediate veterinary attention.

FAILURE TO PASS MANURE ■■■

The fecal material present in the foal's gastrointestinal tract at birth is a sticky, dark, pasty manure, called meconium. Constipation in newborn foals is a fairly common problem (some breeding operations even routinely give enemas to newborns to prevent this) and may be more common in colts than fillies. The foal should be carefully observed for the first 12 to 24 hours to see that it is passing manure frequently and that the manure is not overly dry. Wholly or partially constipated foals will strain often without result. The problem can become serious if not corrected early.

Treatment:

- If the foal shows the above signs of impaction, you can give him an enema, using a commercial preparation such as Fleet's enema (available in drug stores). Be sure to lubricate the tip well with K-Y jelly or Vaseline, insert slowly and gently, never forcing.

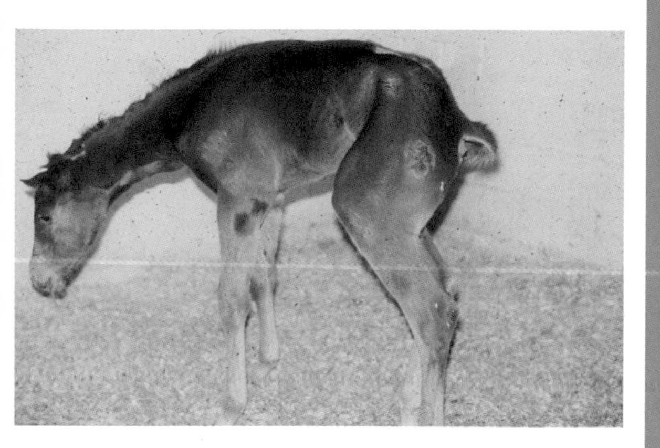

Foals straining to pass manure may have an impaction.

- If the enema meets with minimal or little success, insert several glycerin suppositories into the anus. Wait an hour, and if the foal is still straining unsuccessfully, the enema may be repeated.
- If this is still not successful, the veterinarian should be brought in.

FAILURE TO URINATE ■■■

The foal should also be observed carefully to see that it is urinating normally. Rupture of the bladder can occur during birth. This will result in colic and depression within 24 hours of birth. Prior to that, no urination or passage of only small amounts of urine will be noted. If urination is suspected to be abnormal, get immediate veterinary attention.

WEAK OR DEPRESSED FOALS ■■■

As mentioned above, the normal newborn foal is extremely lively and alert, attentive to all things around

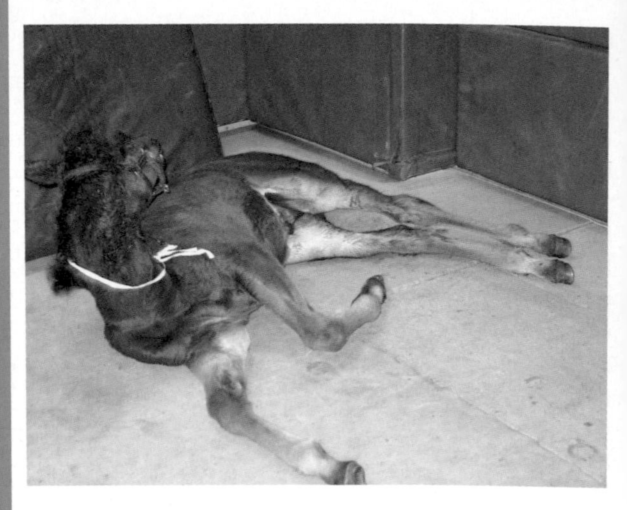

Foals with colic usually lie down and may roll, or roll up onto their backs.

him. His movements are strong, if not always coordinated. Any deviation from this is cause for concern. The problem may be as simple as a low blood sugar or as complicated as a neurological condition. In any case, foals that remain depressed and weak for longer than 20 to 30 minutes after birth should immediately be evaluated by a vet for special care.

HYPOTHERMIA ■■

While even very young foals can survive birth in cold conditions, extremely frigid weather, particularly if combined with a difficult birth, can overcome the foal's capacities, and dangerous hypothermia (subnormal temperature) can set in. The foal's energy stores can be rapidly used up in trying to generate enough body heat. Any foal with a body temperature below 98°F should be warmed with active rubbing, heat lamps or even removal to a heated area until he returns to normal temperature.

LIMB WEAKNESS/DEFORMITIES ■ to ■■

It's common for foals to have the fetlock drop down to the point where it is close to the ground on one or more legs. This weakness in the supporting tendons/ligaments will usually improve quickly over the first three days of life. If it doesn't, get your vet to evaluate the foal. Any fetlock drop extreme enough to cause the joint to actually touch the ground should be evaluated the first day if it doesn't improve within a few hours of the foal being up.

Because of their wide-based stance, especially on the first day of life, the front legs may look like the cannon bones are not positioned straight under the knees. The hind legs may look sickle-hocked (cannon bones angling forward under the body rather than straight up and down), and the points of the hocks from behind often touch or are closer together than normal when standing.

To evaluate how straight a newborn's legs are, you need to look at them when the foal is lying down, before he's bearing any weight. Legs that may look crooked when he's standing can turn out to be perfectly straight when he's down. The best time to check the straightness of the legs is immediately after birth. If you're not sure of what you're seeing, it never hurts to have the vet look at the foal right away. Otherwise, give the foal a few days to strengthen and straighten up before calling the vet.

Any crookedness that actually worsens should be evaluated by the vet immediately.

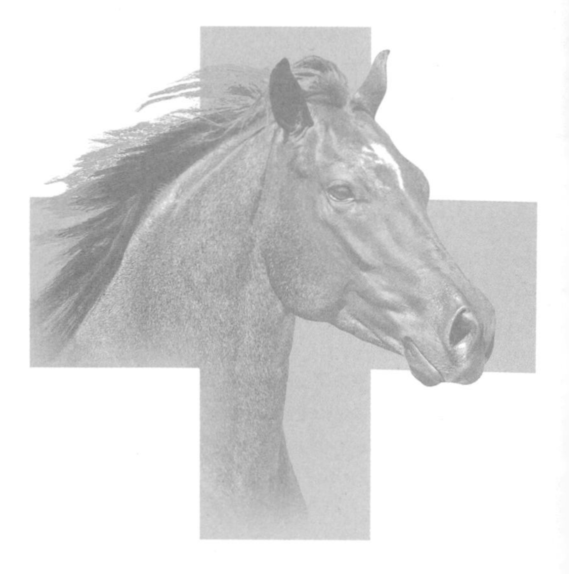

23

DRUG REACTIONS

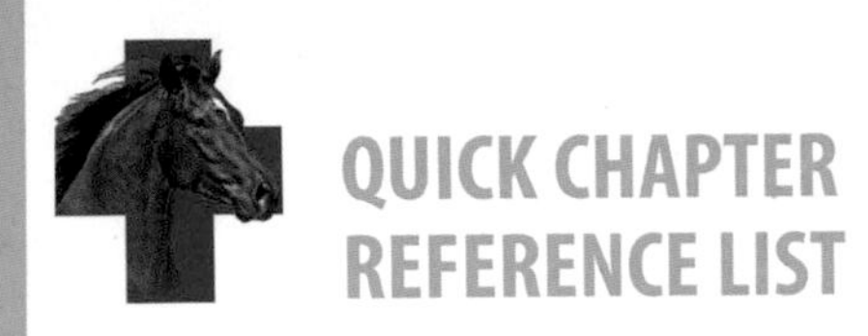

QUICK CHAPTER REFERENCE LIST

LEGEND: ■■■ — NEEDS EMERGENCY ATTENTION; ■■ — SHOULD BE EXAMINED BY A VET; ■ — MAY NEED VETERINARY ADVICE/ATTENTION

℞: PRESCRIPTION DRUG — MUST BE OBTAINED FROM VETERINARIAN OR PRESCRIBED BY A VET — SHOULD NEVER BE ADMINISTERED WITHOUT PRIOR APPROVAL BY A VETERINARIAN.

SOME COMMON DRUG REACTIONS

This chapter does not cover all the possible drug reactions. Some reactions are mild and not true emergencies, and therefore not mentioned. Others are applicable to drugs that should be administered only by a veterinarian, and are acute reactions that would occur while the veterinarian was still present. The drug reactions chosen for inclusion refer to agents that are commonly administered by the horse owner or trainer or are reactions that could occur after the vet has given a drug and left the farm.

TYPES OF DRUG REACTIONS

Specific reactions that may occur with particular drugs are mentioned below. However, any time you give a drug there is the potential for an adverse reaction to occur. Some general types of drug reactions include:

Reactions at intramuscular injection sites

■ to ■■■

All drugs and vaccines given intramuscularly carry the risk of tissue reaction ranging from heat, swelling and pain to actual abscess formation. The reaction can occur within hours or days of the injection. This is most likely to occur with some vaccinations (e.g., flu or Strangles) and with any drug where the label clearly states to give by deep intramuscular injection only.

Intramuscular injection of a drug intended only for intravenous use (e.g., phenylbutazone) is almost guaranteed to produce tissue damage. These reactions, even an

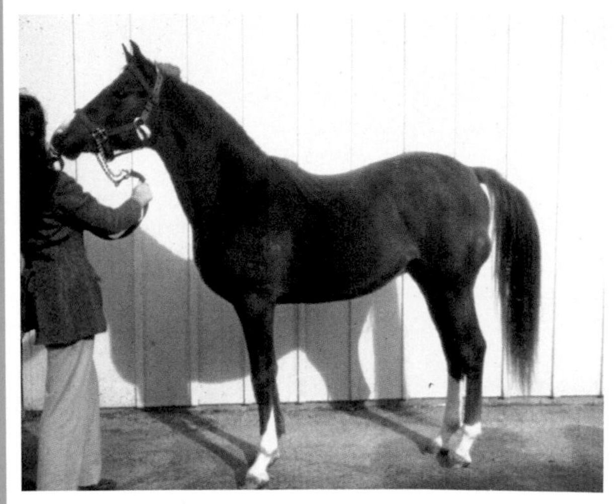

Injection site reactions can occur, like the one on this horse's hindquarters.

abscess, are not emergencies, unless the horse also has a fever or is obviously depressed, although veterinary attention may be needed to open, drain and flush the area. However, if the tissue becomes blackened or develops a peculiar crackling texture when you run your hand over the skin (meaning there is gas in the tissues), immediate veterinary attention is needed. This latter reaction signifies the presence of gas-producing bacteria, which could be fatal.

Damage to veins ■ to ■■

When a drug intended for intravenous injection is deposited into the tissue around the vein rather than in it, a local tissue reaction can occur. The likelihood of this happening depends on both the drug involved and how much ended up outside the vein. The time frame for noticing the reaction and local symptoms are the same as for intramuscular injections above. If you know you gave an injection where some of the drug was deposited outside the vein, apply ice for several hours. (An ice pack can be wrapped on the neck using a polo wrap.) Keep the horse cross-tied with the head elevated but in a comfortable position, and call your vet for any further instructions.

If the neck, throat and head on the side of the missed injection begin to swell, get the vet out to examine the horse immediately. This indicates a complete obstruction of the vein and if severe, may interfere with breathing and/or swallowing.

Hives ■

Hives are a rather nonspecific allergic/hyper-sensitivity reaction that may occur after the use of any drug, but are rare with the first exposure to a drug. The reaction can be stopped with use of corticosteroids but hives do not usually require treatment other than avoiding any further use of the drug, and they will resolve on their own. A horse that develops hives, though, should be watched closely over the next several hours to make sure the reaction doesn't progress to breathing difficulties. Internal edema of the throat may be occurring at the same time.

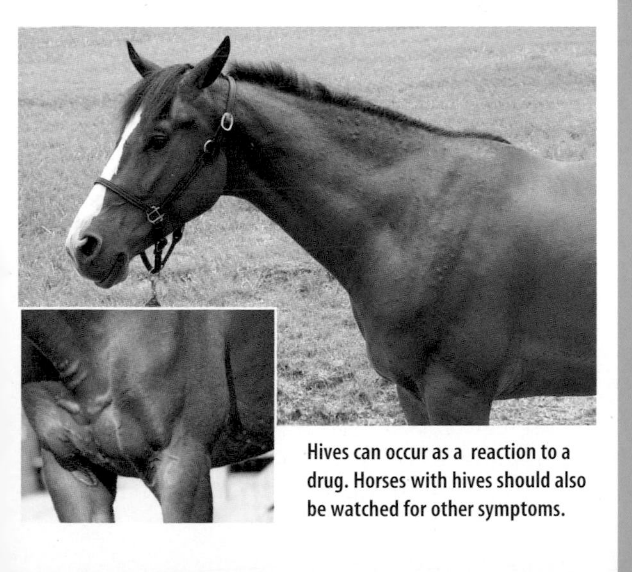

Hives can occur as a reaction to a drug. Horses with hives should also be watched for other symptoms.

Skin reactions ■ to ■■

In rare cases, sensitivity to a drug may cause a skin reaction such as blister formation, diffuse swelling, cracking, oozing of fluid through the skin. Reaction may be widespread or limited to only some parts of the body. Contact your vet immediately if any unexplained skin problem develops when your horse is on any drug.

Clotting abnormalities may also occur. Treatment involves stopping the drug and administering corticosteroids.

Anaphylaxis ■■■

Anaphylaxis is a term used to describe any severe drug reaction. Within seconds or minutes of administering a drug, the horse will show agitation/trembling, elevated heart rate, heavy breathing, sweating and possibly collapse. Swelling of the throat may occur rapidly and interfere with breathing. Hives may appear. Anaphylaxis is usually treated with epinephrine (see below under tranquilizers).

ANTIBIOTICS

Procaine penicillin ■

Some horses develop an "allergy" (reaction) to procaine penicillin (the intramuscular form of penicillin) characterized by twitching, agitation and excitability within 5 to 15 minutes of administration, although in some cases the reaction may begin before the injection is even completed. It's unclear whether this is a true penicillin allergy or a reaction to procaine. It may also be from too rapid an absorption of the drug secondary to direct injection into a vessel or to injection into a muscular site previously used for multiple injections where tissue damage resulted in a greater than normal blood supply. In any case, there is no specific treatment called for, and the reaction will pass on its own with the horse starting to come out of it usually within 10 minutes or so. He should be back to normal, but possibly still looking depressed or shaky, within a half an hour. However, that horse should not receive any further procaine penicillin.

Tetracycline ■

Tetracycline is given intravenously by the veterinarian, usually to treat a lung infection. Horses carrying a salmonella infection may develop a full-blown case of salmonella diarrhea during the course of treatment with tetracycline. If diarrhea to any degree develops, isolate the horse and alert the veterinarian.

Sulfa drugs ■■

Although rare, horses with low-level renal function problems may have trouble handling sulfa drugs and may develop renal failure. This should be considered if a horse on sulfas develops depression or decreased appetite or generally seems ill for no apparent reason. Diagnosis requires blood tests. Call the vet if any horse receiving sulfa drugs (or any drug) begins to look worse or develops new symptoms.

-mycin drugs (Gentamicin, Streptomycin, Amikacin etc.) ■■

These can cause renal failure in high doses or when given to very ill animals. See sulfa antibiotics, above.

TRANQUILIZERS ■■

Accidental injection of tranquilizers into an artery instead of a vein can cause severe reactions. The promazine group (e.g., acepromazine) given intra-arterially may cause profound sedation and a rapid drop in blood pressure, even collapse. When xylazine (Rompun) is given into an artery, extreme agitation occurs.

To avoid this, intravenous injections should be given as low down in the neck as possible, as the vein and artery are close together in the upper neck. Better yet, **any injection of tranquilizer given without a veterinarian present should be given intramuscularly unless the caregiver is experienced and confident in giving intravenous injections.**

In the event of collapse following xylazine injection, give epinephrine, 1:1,000 strength, 4 to 8 cc. in muscle or under the skin. Follow the directions on the bottle. Carefully read them in advance of any such emergency. **Epinephrine should not be given to a horse that has had acepromazine**, however.

DEWORMERS ■ to ■■

All deworming preparations are capable of causing the horse to go off feed and even to show mild signs of colic. This should resolve in a day or so, but it is wise to withhold grain in horses that have gone off feed or show mild colic signs, and to check their feet routinely for signs of laminitis. Laminitis was more of a problem with the older preparations for bots that had to be administered by stomach tube than with today's paste formulas. Refer to Chapter 7, page 73.

B VITAMINS ■■

Injectable B vitamins are sometimes administered by trainers, either alone or in combination with intravenous fluids, to combat stress during periods of heavy competition. However, there is a fairly high incidence of horses having adverse reactions, ranging from trembling and weakness to collapse and even death. Reactions can occur even in a horse that has previously received injectable B vitamins without any problems. High doses given rapidly are most likely to cause the problem, but there is no 100-percent safe way to inject B vitamins in horses. Giving a test dose of approximately 1/3 the total dose by the intramuscular route and observing the horse for 15 minutes will pick up some of the horses that are hypersensitive, but it is not a guarantee against reactions. The best solution is not to give injectable B vitamins, or to have the veterinarian administer them. In the event of collapse, use epinephrine (see Tranquilizers, page 227).

Even oral B-vitamin supplementation may cause problems. Large doses of thiamine can cause tranquilization. Niacin or even multiple B supplements in large doses can cause excitement. You can call the vet to be on the safe side, but if the tranquilization is caused by vitamin-B supplementation, there's nothing you can do except wait for it to wear off.

PHENYLBUTAZONE AND OTHER ANTI-INFLAMMATORY DRUGS ■■

These agents are capable of causing irritation — even ulceration — of the gastrointestinal tract, which in turn results in decreased appetite, particularly for grain, and even signs of mild colic. Individual increased sensitivity or an underlying irritation, (e.g., bots in the stomach) may results in problems a short time after starting treatment. Generally, however, this is a complication of long-term and/or high-dose therapy. Giving phenylbutazone at the same time as hay can slow absorption of the drug so that it is still being absorbed when the next dose is given, resulting in an overdose. You can try giving the drug only after the horse has eaten, mixing it in 30cc of Milk of Magnesia to make a slurry to deliver by oral syringe. If this does not alleviate the symptoms, discontinue the drug.

REPRODUCTIVE DRUGS ■ to ■■

Prostaglandin is sometimes given to mares to shorten the time it will take for them to come back into season. This drug can cause sweating, elevated pulse/breathing rate and abdominal discomfort. However, these are side effects of the drug, not a true drug reaction, and require no treatment.

HCG, human chorionic gonadotropin, is used to cause a mare with a large follicle to ovulate within 24 hours, so that breeding can be timed to deliver the sperm close to ovulation. Because this hormone is not the same as equine hormones, many mares develop antibodies to it after repeated uses. Reactions usually occur anywhere from half an hour to a few hours after injection and include hives, depression, swelling and edema. These reactions are usually self-limiting and will begin to reverse within a few hours. Call the vet to describe the reaction and get advice regarding whether treatment (usually corticosteroids) is indicated. Any mare that looks like she is developing trouble breathing should be seen immediately.

Precautions

Serious drug reactions require immediate, on-the-spot attention within minutes. If you routinely give drugs yourself, go over the list of medications with your vet so that you fully understand the possible reactions and how to respond to them. **If you get into trouble with a serious drug reaction, you won't have time to wait for your vet to get there.** Your vet may decide it's a good idea for you to keep epinephrine and/or a corticosteroid drug on hand in the event of a reaction. If this is the case, make sure you fully understand how to give the drug, and the appropriate dosage.

Troubleshooting after the vet leaves

Reactions can vary widely depending on the specific drug involved, the severity of the reaction, and the differences in how long it should normally take any drug-related problem to resolve. Be sure you get detailed instructions from your vet regarding what you can expect to see and in what time frame, and when you need to call her back.

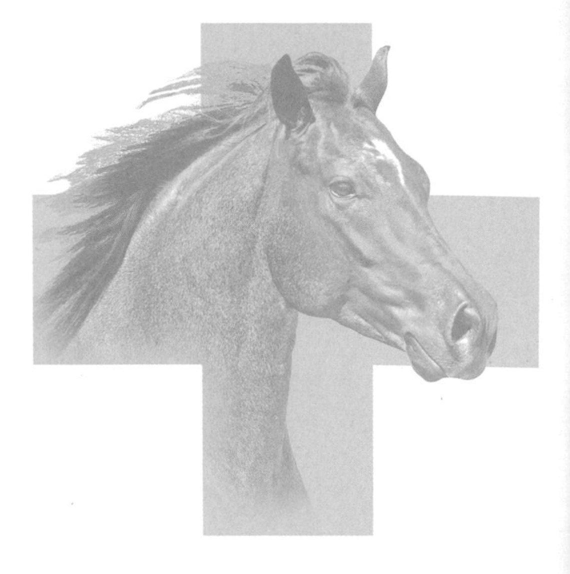

24
REFERENCE

REFERENCE

NORMAL VALUES FOR A HORSE AT REST — TPR (Temperature, Pulse, and Respiration)

Temperature: 98°F to 100°F
Pulse: 44 beats per minute
(Range high 20s to low 40s)
Respiration: 8 to 16 breaths per minute

Weather conditions will affect values (i.e., higher on hot days). Excitement and fear will quickly elevate pulse and respiration, which will just as quickly return to normal when the animal is quiet. Foals will have higher values than adult horses.

DESCRIBING HORSE ANATOMY

Knowing the names of parts of the horse is a help when communicating with the vet on the phone.

The illustration below shows the relative terms that are sometimes used in describing the location of a wound. For instance, proximal to something means closer to it, distal means farther away, and caudal means facing the rear.

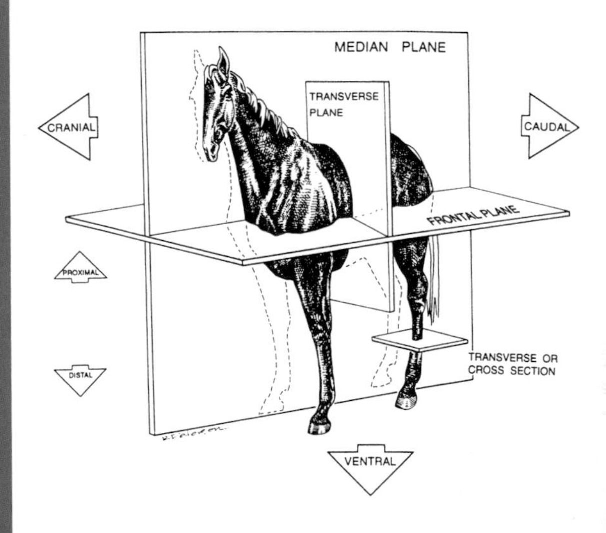

Points of the horse

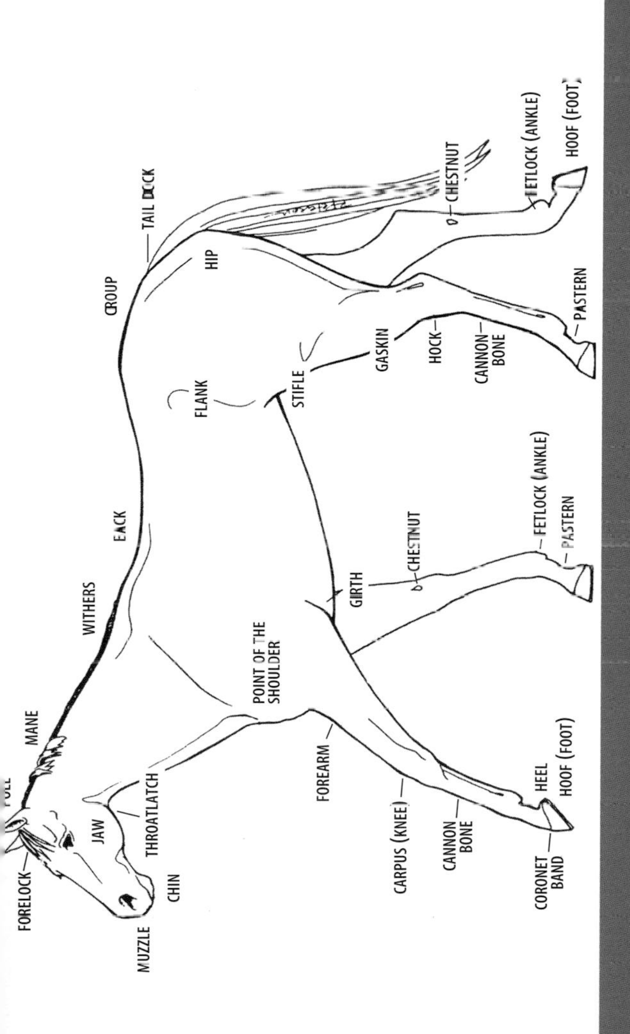

Points of the horse — Front

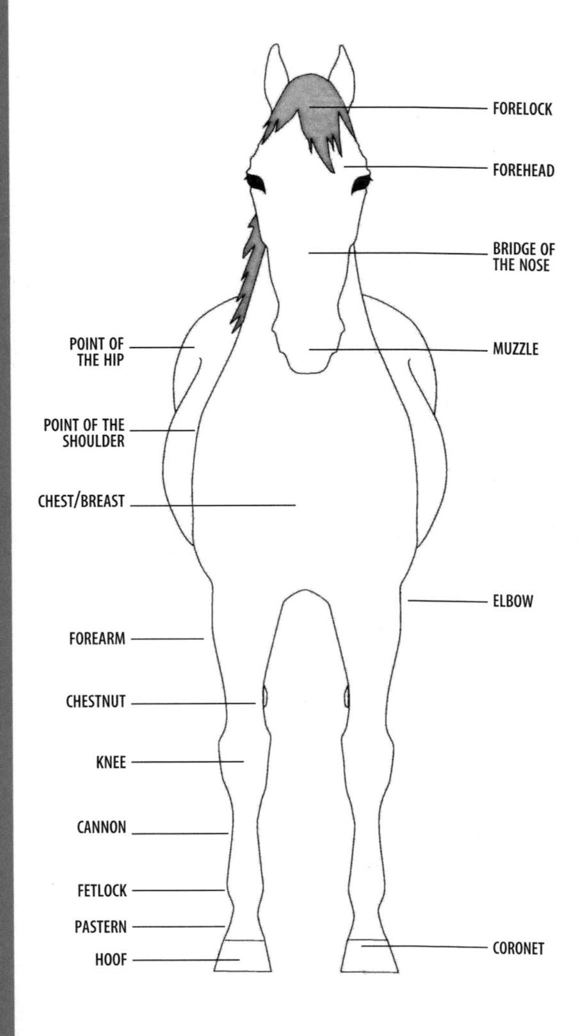

Points of the horse — Back

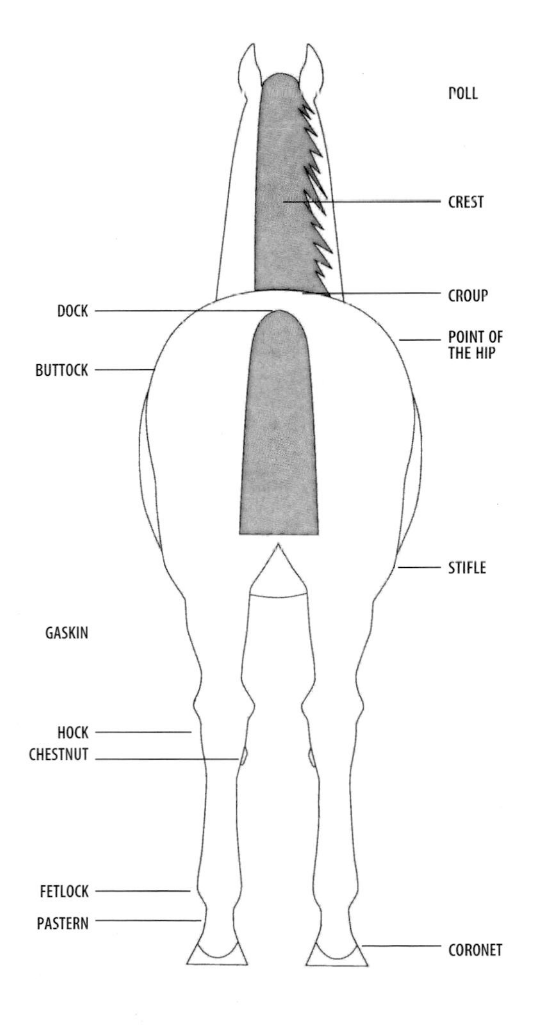

SIGNS OF EFFECTIVE TRANQUILIZATION

The horse must be observed from a distance. Any horse may be temporarily aroused to a state of alertness when handled. The horse can still kick, strike, etc., when tranquilized. However, his reactions will be much slower unless suddenly startled, and it will usually take more stimulus to cause the undesired reaction.

Most common signs of effective tranquilization:

- Head held low
- Drooping eyelids
- Drooping lower lip and/or ears
- Penis relaxed/hanging
- Wide-based stance in front
- Noisy breathing *

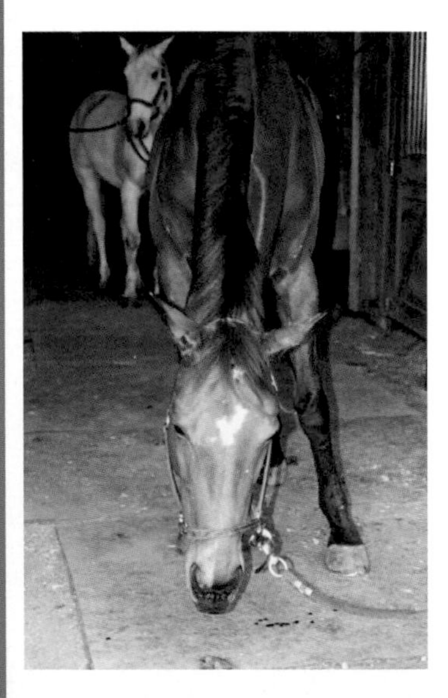

** Not a necessary sign — indicates moderate to heavy tranquilization with partial paralysis of the throat. Remove hay, feed, and water until breathing returns to normal.*

Tranquilized horses can suddenly "wake up" and kick or strike without warning.

SIGNS OF SHOCK

Shock is a body-wide reaction to a severe injury, illness, or metabolic problem. Heavy blood loss, severe dehydration, electrolyte disturbances, extensive wounds, and severe pain can all cause symptoms of shock. Treatment is primarily directed at solving the underlying problem. It's also important to put the horse in a quiet location where he will not be disturbed/excited, blanket him lightly if he is shivering, and avoid giving any drugs until the veterinarian has evaluated the horse.

Signs of shock:

- Weakness
- Trembling
- Depression
- Cold ears
- Cold lower legs
- Rapid, weak pulse (over 50 beats per minute)
- Pale mucous membranes
- Increased capillary refill time (over 2 seconds)
- Decreased urinary output
- Obvious sweating or a damp feeling to the body.

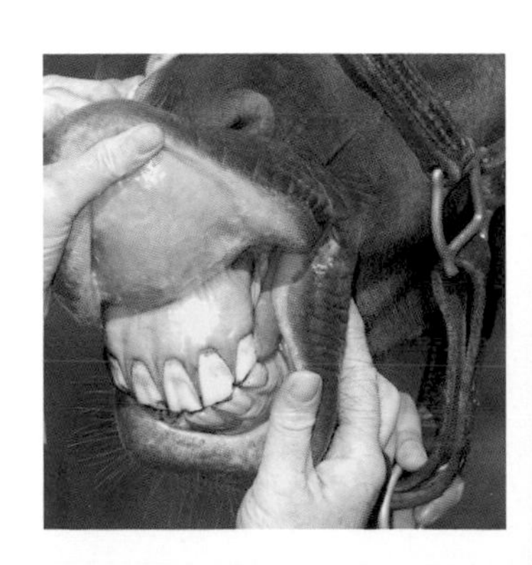

To check a horse's mucous membrane color, raise his lips and note the color of his gums.

ALTERNATIVE THERAPIES

There is a growing tendency toward the use of "natural" products, rather than manufactured drugs. When using natural remedies, keep in mind that they are still drugs, not foods, and have the potential for side effects. Here's a guideline regarding their use.

DRUG CATEGORY

Anti-inflammatory/analgesics (e.g., phenylbutazone, flunixin) for musculoskeletal problems

- **Alternative: Devil's Claw** – 2,000 to 3,000 mg one to three times daily in the feed.
  Comments: *Effect = 1 to 2 grams of phenylbutazone*
- **Alternative: Boswellia** – 1,200 mg one to three times daily in the feed.
  Comments: *Effect = 1 to 2 grams of phenylbutazone, but it may take 2+ days to be effective.*
- **Alternative: Ice**
  Comments: *Topical cooling is one of the most effective ways to block pain and inflammation.*
- **Alternative: Arnica** – topical applied several times/day.
  Comments: *Very effective topical herb for pain and inflammation.*

Tranquilizers

- **Alternative: None**
  Comments: *Not effective enough for the emergency situation.*

Colic/abdominal pain medications

- **Alternative: Not recommended**
  Comments: *Although some remedies are potent enough to influence abdominal pain, they will interfere with diagnosis and may react with necessary drugs.*

DRUG NOTES

SOME COMMONLY USED DRUGS

Note: *These are all prescription drugs and should never be used without specific instructions, including dosages, from your vet. Never assume that a drug you used in a similar situation with another horse is appropriate for your current condition. If you do use a drug before you can talk to your vet, always tell him/her exactly what you have used and how much. If the horse has to be trailered to a hospital for treatment, a complete list of drugs the horse has received at home, from both caretakers and the farm vet, should go with the horse to the hospital — including the drug name, dosage, and time of treatment.*

- **Acepromazine:** Tranquilizer. Wide individual variations in how sensitive horses are to the effects. May cause dangerous loss of balance. May cause dangerous lowering of blood pressure.
- **Atropine eye ointment.** Dilates the pupil to minimize spasm/pain and help prevent scarring inside the eye. May cause colic in sensitive horses.
- **Dexamethasone** injection, pills, or powder. Corticosteroid anti-inflammatory. Used for shock, allergic reactions, and severe inflammation. May cause laminitis in sensitive horses. Never use if laminitis is a possible diagnosis. Reduces the ability to fight infections. Will elevate blood sugar and may cause increased drinking and urinating.
- **Doxycycline** pills. Antibiotic. Prolonged use may lead to fungal infections. May cause diarrhea/colitis. Allergic reactions are possible.

℞: PRESCRIPTION DRUG — MUST BE OBTAINED FROM VETERINARIAN OR PRESCRIBED BY A VET — SHOULD NEVER BE ADMINISTERED WITHOUT PRIOR APPROVAL BY A VETERINARIAN.

- **Flunixin meglumine** (Banamine). Injectable, granules, paste. Nonsteroidal anti-inflammatory. Used for fever and muscular, eye, joint, tendon/ligament and other soft tissue pain. Fairly effective for colic pain. High doses or prolonged use may cause ulcers in the mouth or intestinal tract.
- **Gentamicin** (Gentocin). Injectable. Antibiotic. Prolonged use may lead to fungal infections. May cause diarrhea/colitis Allergic reactions are possible. May cause kidney damage or deafness with prolonged use. Never give orally.
- **Penicillin.** Injectable. Antibiotic. Prolonged use may lead to fungal infections. May cause diarrhea/colitis. Allergic reactions are possible. One of the most common allergies. Never give orally. **Never inject into a vein**.
- **Phenylbutazone.** ("Bute") Injectable, pills, powder, paste. Nonsteroidal anti-inflammatory. Used for fever and muscular, eye, joint, tendon/ligament, and other soft tissue pain. Poorly effective for colic pain. High doses or prolonged use may cause ulcers in the mouth or intestinal tract. **The injectable form should only be given intravenously**. Phenylbutazone causes severe reactions if injected outside a vein. Oral forms of phenylbutazone are also available.
- **Trimethoprim/sulfa.** Injection, paste, or pills. Antibiotic. Prolonged use may lead to fungal infections. May cause diarrhea/colitis. Allergic reactions are possible.
- **Xylazine** (Rompun). Tranquilizer. Wide individual variations in how sensitive horses are to the effects. May cause dangerous loss of balance. May cause dangerous lowering of blood pressure.

HERB/DRUG INTERACTIONS

The following is a list of some commonly used Western herbs with potential drug interactions important in a first-aid setting. This is not a complete list. As a general rule, when an herb has been given to a horse for a specific reason, such as calming, you must assume the potential is there for interaction with drugs that have similar effects, like tranquilizers or anesthetics.

Key:

A may interact with anesthetics or tranquilizers
B may lower blood pressure
C* may interfere with clotting
H hormonal effects
HB may raise blood pressure
I immune system stimulation, avoid in horses with allergies

** Most herbs marked C should not be combined with any nonsteroidal anti-inflammatory drugs, including aspirin, or with drugs that directly influence clotting (heparin, warfarin)*

List of Herbs:

Angelica (C)
Astragalus (I)
Black Cohosh (H)
Cat's Claw (B, C, H)
Chamomile (A, C)
Don Quai (C)
Echinacea (I)
Feverfew (C)
Garlic (C)
Ginger (C)
Ginkgo (C)
Ginsengs (C, HB)
Gynostemma (B, C)
Hawthorn (B, C)
Kava Kava (A)
Licorice (H, HB)
Red Clover (H)
Salvia (C)
Valerian (A)

PREVENTION AND TREATMENT OF ACUTE FLARE-UPS

Certainly not all emergencies can be avoided, but there are some chronic conditions that always pose risks of acute flare-ups. Below are some brief suggestions for both spotting a worsening of the condition and helping to minimize those acute flare-ups.

LAMINITIS

- Recurrent bouts of laminitis are often the result of hormonal problems (Cushing's disease, insulin resistance), so have the horse tested for these conditions and treat/manage appropriately.
- Avoid grazing spring and fall pastures in horses with a history of grass laminitis.
- Never let the horse go too long between trims, and make sure to keep the toes short and the heels low.
- Do not allow free exercise, or ride the horse, when he's being treated with a pain-relieving/anti-inflammatory drug.

IMPACTION COLIC

- Have the teeth checked and attended to at regular intervals (every 6 to 12 months).
- Deworm regularly, including at least once a year for tapeworms.
- If problems persist in an older horse despite good chewing, consider feeding complete feeds, preferably moistened.

- Monitor water intake carefully to be sure a hay-fed horse is drinking 8 to 10 gallons of water in cool weather, 2 to 3 times that amount in hot weather.
- If water intake is low, add salt directly to the food — 1 oz./day in cold weather, 2 oz./day when hot, plus offer a salt block or loose salt

HEAT-RELATED PROBLEMS

- Never work the horse hard in the heat when there's been a sudden increase in temperature.
- Monitor water intake and provide generous salt, as above.
- Remember dark-colored horses heat up quicker than light-colored.
- Never ask for unusually hard or long work-outs in the heat.
- Stop or slow down when you see signs of fatigue — labored breathing, tripping, stumbling, heavy on the forehand.

ERU (EQUINE RECURRENT UVEITIS, PERIODIC OPHTHALMIA, MOON BLINDNESS)

- Learn the early warning signs of tearing, avoidance of light, graying of the cornea.
- Use fly masks when turned out in the daytime.
- Never stop treatment abruptly after an acute flare-up.
- Follow instructions to the letter regarding timing, dosages, and duration of therapy.
- Deworm at least twice a year to lessen chances of onchocerciasis (connective tissue infection with the larval stages of onchocherca).
- Isolate from cattle, practice good rodent control, and keep horse away from natural water sources to minimize exposure to Leptospirosis.

LAMENESS/ARTHRITIS

- Keep feet properly trimmed and balanced at all times.
- Use common sense in working horses too long, in mud/sand/deep footing or on very hard surfaces.
- Allow as much turn out time as possible.
- Keep to a schedule of regular formal exercise.
- Always do a slow warm up (e.g., walking, slow trot for 10 minutes).
- Use joint nutraceuticals (chondroitin, glucosamine, perna mussel, hyaluronic acid).
- Apply ice to known problem areas immediately after any hard work.
- If the horse always starts out stiff, consider a brisk liniment massage to the area before work.

COPD/HEAVES

- Feed generous levels of vitamin C, vitamin E and selenium year round.
- Know the common triggers and aggravating factors and how to avoid them (poor circulation in barn, dust in hay/grain/straw, grain allergies).
- If the horse has a known high-risk time of year, talk to your veterinarian about starting medications before the horse gets into trouble in hopes of avoiding a major flare-up.

25

PROCEDURES

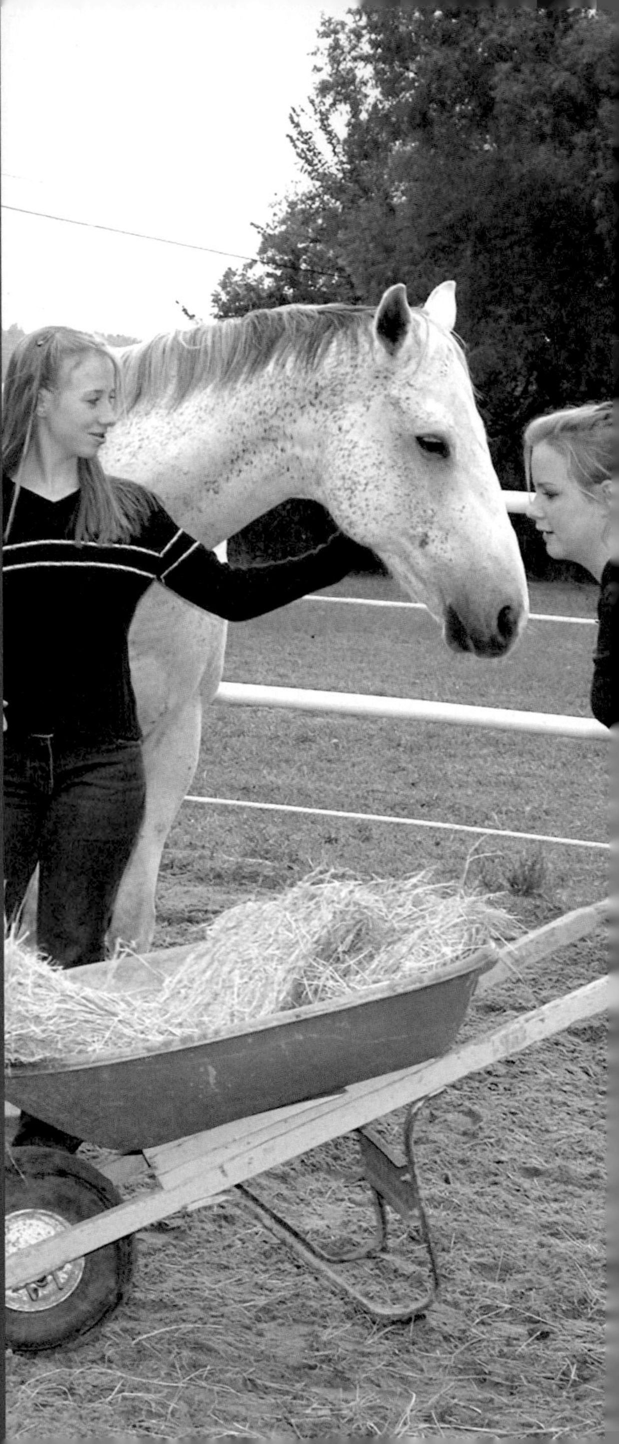

PROCEDURES

READING VITAL SIGNS

The horse's temperature, pulse, and respiration are referred to as his "vital signs," since they reflect the general health of some of his vital systems (heart, lungs, immune system, temperature regulation). They also, nonspecifically, show whether the horse is distressed. They are important barometers of how a problem is progressing — becoming more abnormal if the condition worsens and returning toward normal as the horse improves. Whenever you suspect a problem, recording the horse's temperature, pulse, and respiration (TPR) should be among the first steps you take.

TEMPERATURE

Take the horse's temperature rectally, using a special horse thermometer, which is larger and stronger than thermometers used for people. Human digital thermometers may not give accurate readings in horses since the short tip does not enter the rectum far enough.

To prevent losing the thermometer into the rectum, attach a string to the hole located at the end of the thermometer and from there to a clothespin or other suitable clip. The thermometer may then be safely clipped to the tail hairs. Cool water, petroleum jelly or other gel lubricant may be used to ease insertion.

- Stand to the side of the horse, close to his body. Do not stand behind him.
- Move his tail to one side so you can see the anus, and insert the thermometer.

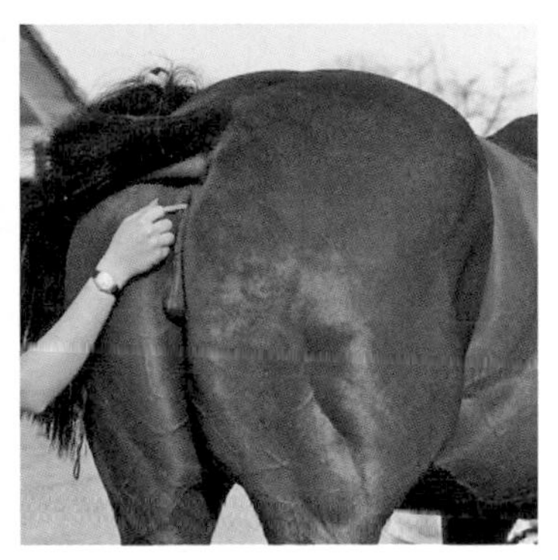

- Leave the thermometer in for approximately 2 minutes for an accurate reading (try to avoid inserting it into fecal material — that will give false readings).

Normal temperatures are anywhere between 98° and 100° (rarely as high as 100.5 or 101°) for an adult horse at rest, depending on individual variation and the weather conditions. Normal temperature for foals is up to 101°F.

PULSE

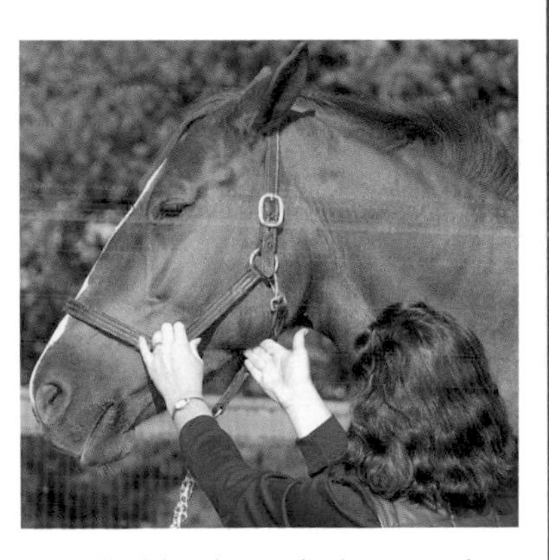

The pulse is taken by gently pressing the fingertips against an artery that is close to the surface of the skin. The best location for this is along the lower edge of the cheek muscle or jaw. The blood vessels there can be easily felt rolling under the skin. Wait until you can feel the pulse clearly and then count the number of beats per minute (or beats per 15 seconds and multiply by four).

Normal pulse is anywhere from the high 20s to the low 40s, depending on how excited the horse is at the time, as well as the weather and his level of fitness.

RESPIRATION

The respiratory rate is taken by observing the movement of the ribs (out as he inhales, in as he exhales) and counting the number of breaths per minute, as described above for pulse. Nostril movement is not reliable. If you have trouble seeing the chest move, place a hand on the horse's body so that you can feel it too.

Normal respiration is approximately 8 to 16 breaths per minute, with the rate being influenced by the same factors as described above for temperature and pulse.

"CAP REFILL"

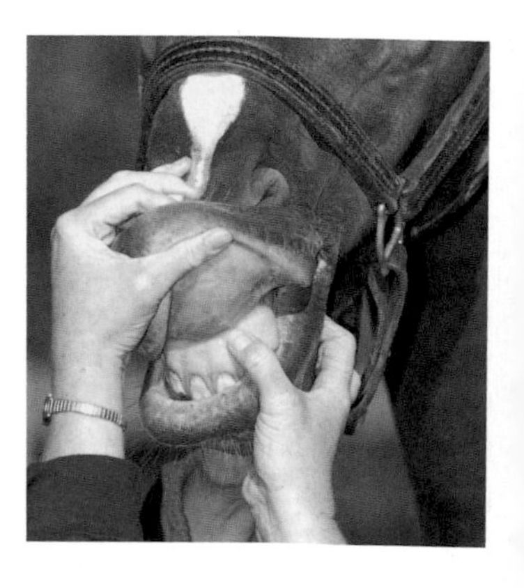

Lift the horse's top lip, and press a finger against his gums. That will force blood out of the capillaries in that spot and turn the spot white. Notice how quickly color returns to the spot. Normal refill has the pink color returning within two seconds. Longer than that means the horse is dealing with dehydration, shock, or some other problem. Notify your veterinarian immediately.

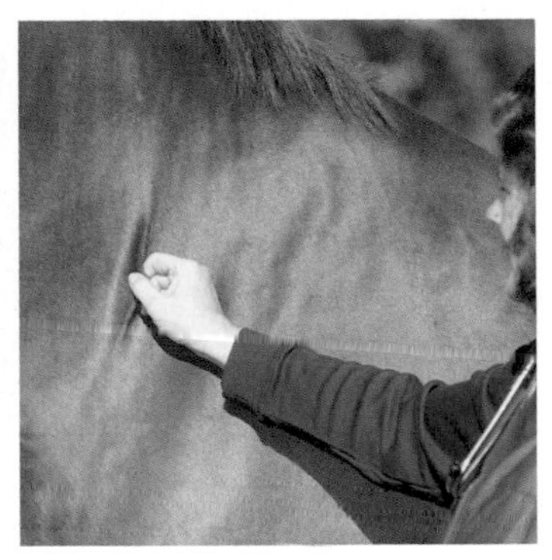

SKIN ELASTICITY TEST FOR DEHYDRATION

Grasp the skin at the base of the horse's neck above his shoulder into a fold, then release it. If the horse is not dehydrated, the skin should spring back into place. (Try this with the skin on the back of your hand.)

If the skin stays folded or returns to normal slowly, then the horse is dealing with some degree of dehydration. Provide water, if the horse is able to drink, and notify your veterinarian.

CHECK FEET FOR HEAT

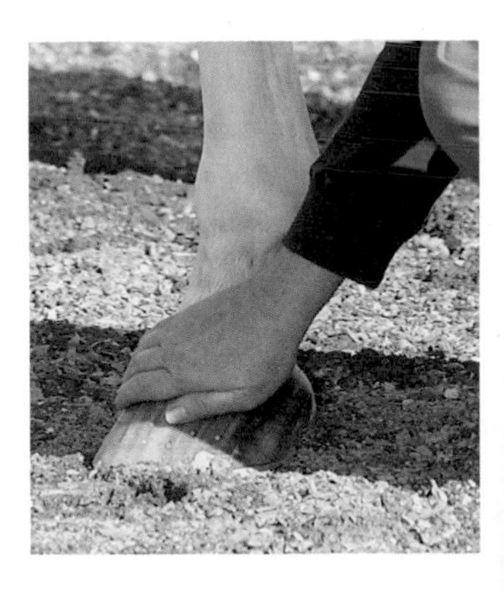

Place your hand over the front of the horse's hoof, and hold it there for two seconds. Compare that to the temperature felt on his other feet. You may have to compare it to a well horse to see what normal is likely to be. Feet feeling inappropriately hot or cold, and feet feeling a different temperature than the others should be reported to the vet immediately.

TWITCHING THE HORSE

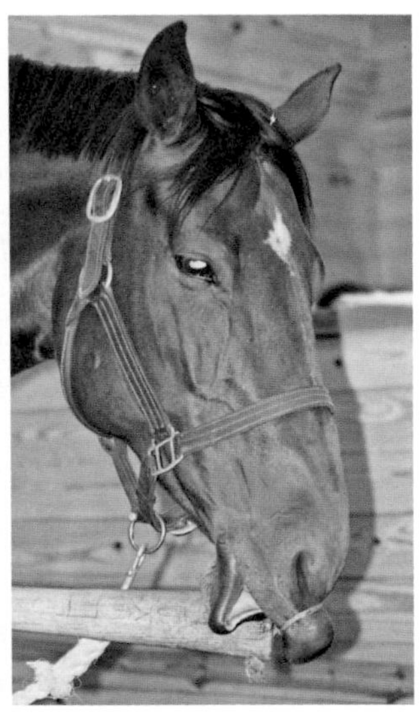

Although it seems unusually cruel to some people, twitching is a basic and often quite necessary method of restraint, particularly when dealing with an injured and/or frightened horse.

While it would seem that twitches of any sort should cause pain, it has been shown that the horse's respiratory and heart rates actually decrease when he is twitched, much as if under the effect of a tranquilizer, and not at all as would be expected if the horse was in considerable pain.

Great care should be taken when using a twitch. Do not stand in front of the horse, as some horses almost reflexively strike a foot forward. Stand on the same side as a helper or someone going to treat the horse.

There are several types of twitches, and their application differs slightly. Basically, hold the horse's halter with one hand. Grasp a generous portion of the horse's top lip/nose with the other. Don't twist the nose. Let go of the halter, and slip the loop of the twitch over the hand and onto the nose.

If you're using a rope or chain twitch, which is basically a loop of rope or chain attached to a wooden handle, then continue to hold the horse's nose while you turn the twitch to tighten the loop around the nose, just snug enough to keep the loop from slipping off. Alternately, a second person can tighten the twitch. Once snug, apply sufficient constant twist to the handle to prevent it from loosening and falling off — the amount of pressure needed to be decided by how much resistance the horse is giving. Use as little pressure as is necessary.

If you're using a "humane horse twitch," which is two shaped aluminum rods hinged together, then you'd open the twitch, slip the shaped part near the hinge over the horse's nose, then squeeze the handles enough to close the twitch onto the horse's nose. The twitch can be held by an assistant (best way) or the string at the end wrapped around the handles and clipped to the halter ring.

The person controlling the twitch should then also take over the lead shank and position himself on the same side as the person doing treatments.

BANDAGING

ROUTINE STANDING LEG WRAP

- Wrap a quilted cotton wrap so that the beginning and the end lie across the front or side of the cannon bone, not on the tendons.
- Tuck three inches of the outer, elastic (polo) wrap under the cotton wrap one-third to halfway up the leg.
- Angle the wrap downward, and carefully wrap the bandage around the leg, keeping the pressure even and avoiding all wrinkles.
- As you bandage, overlap the previous wrap for a width of 1/3 to 1/2 the width of the wrap. Work your way down the leg. If desired, at the back of the ankle (fetlock) you can make one or two loops that travel under the sesamoids and back of the joint, to provide extra support and relief from strain.
- Change direction smoothly, avoiding wrinkles, and work back up the leg to finish the wrap at the top of the leg.

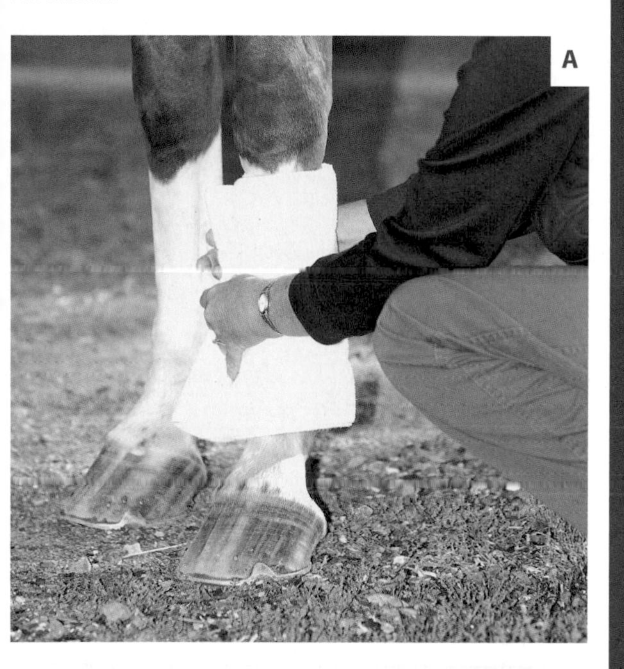
A

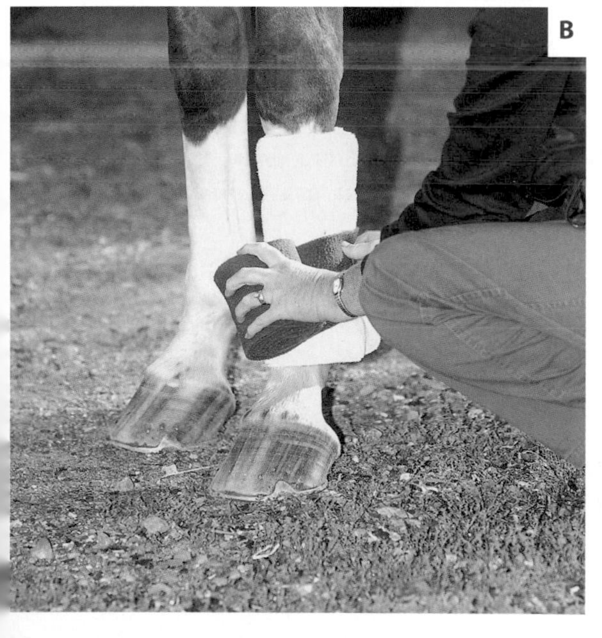
B

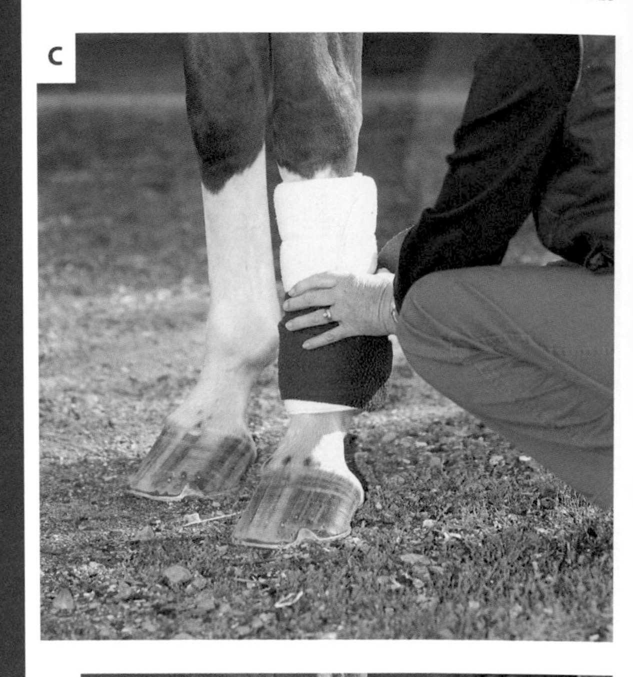
C

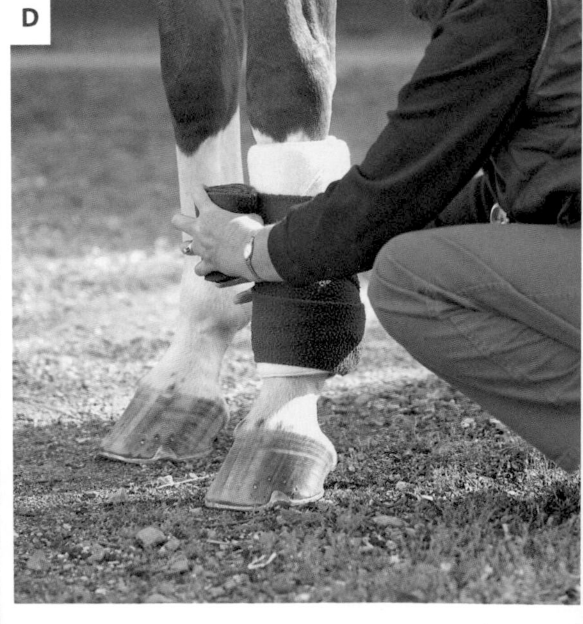
D

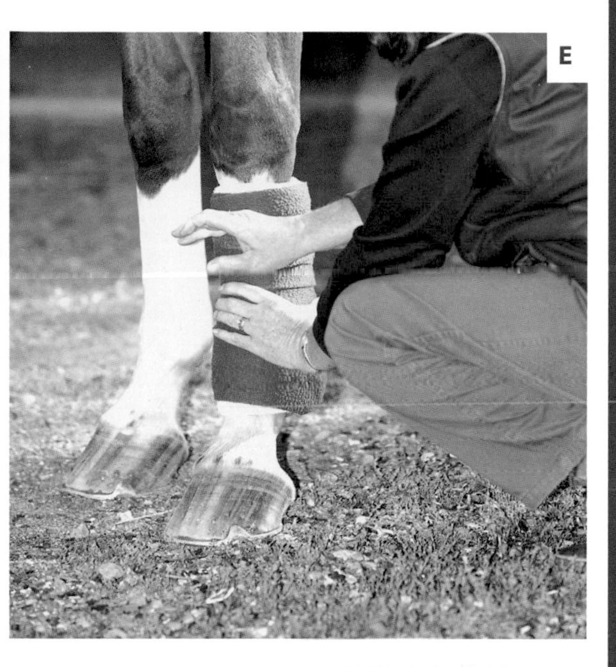
E

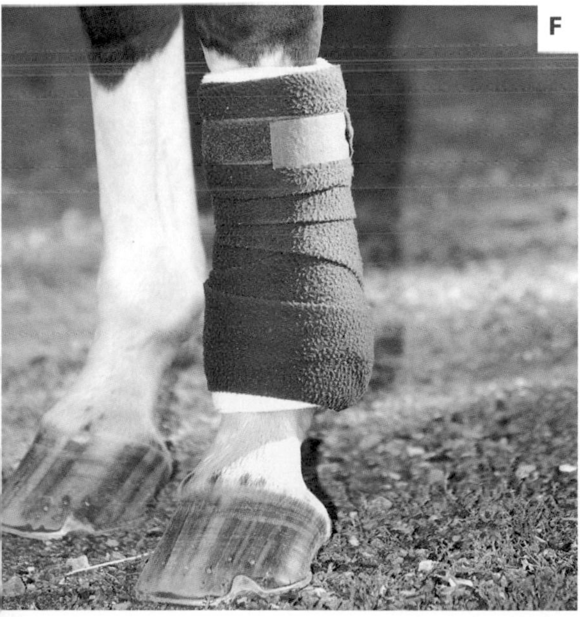
F

FIGURE-OF-EIGHT LEG WRAP

The figure-of-eight leg wrap is another way to apply pressure across the knee and is also useful for the hock. Do not apply this bandage so tightly that the skin is indented.

- Begin the wrap by encircling the leg once or twice below the hock (or knee).
- Next, angle the wrap up across the front of the joint, from inside to outside.
- Next, make two loops above the joint, then begin downward again, crossing the joint from inside to outside to make an "X".
- Repeat the crisscrossing several times, making loops above and below the joint as well as needed to stabilize the wrap and keep it from slipping down.
- Finish the wrap, either above or below the joint, with a straight, encircling loop.

Note that when doing the hock, the point of the hock is left free to allow the leg to move. Similarly, when doing a knee, the prominent accessory carpal bone at the back of the knee is left free. Be careful not to apply this bandage too tight. Use just enough tension that the bandage will not flip.

FOR THE HOCK

A

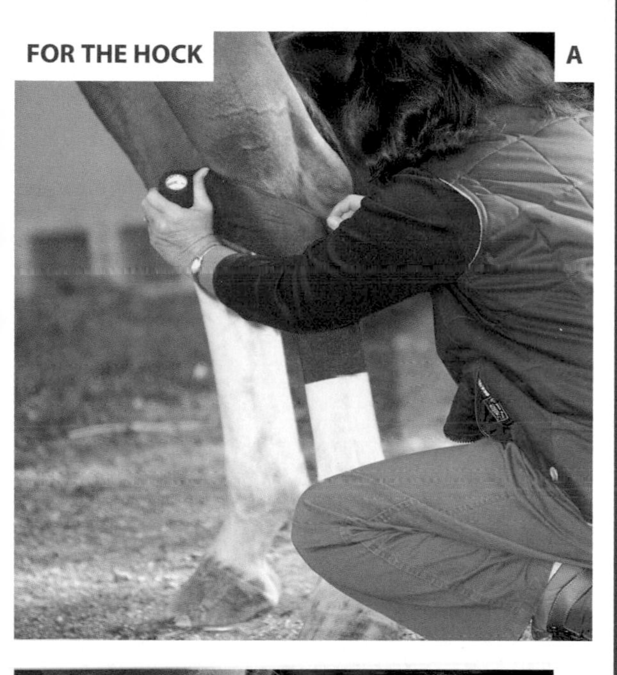

B

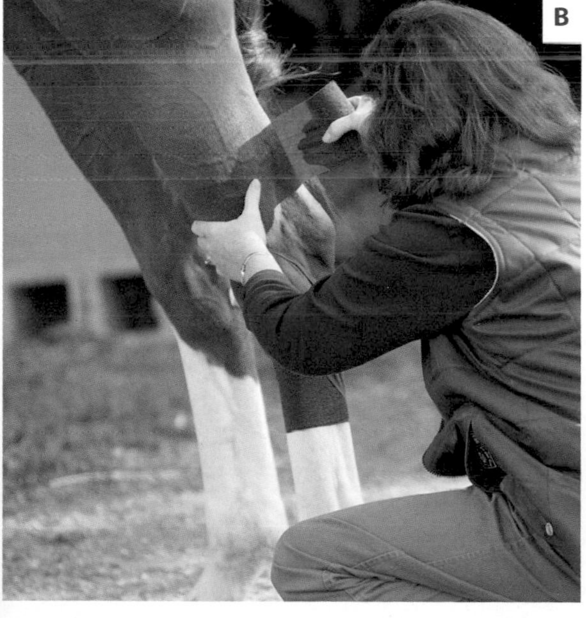

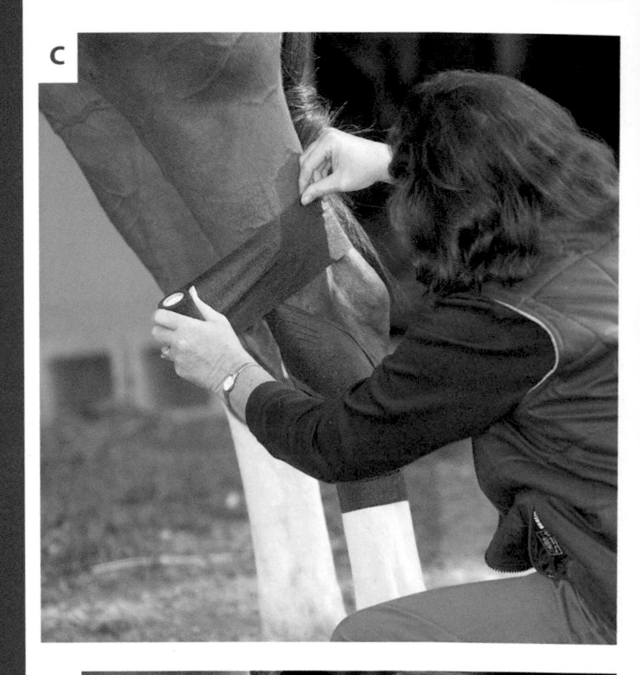
C

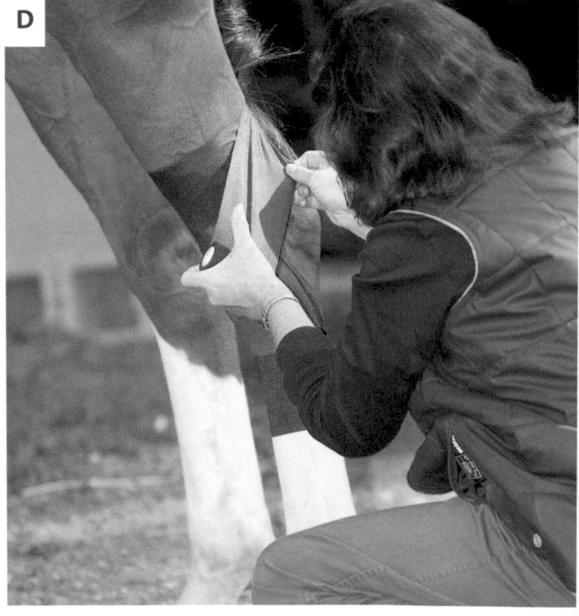
D

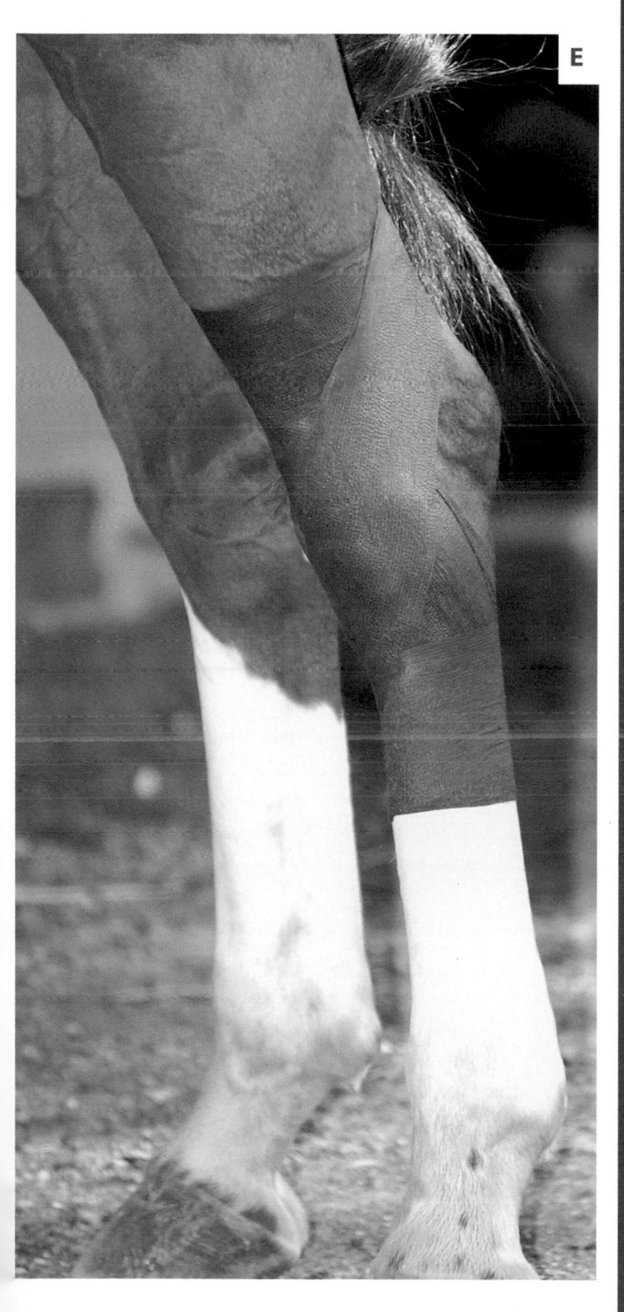
E

FOR THE KNEE

A

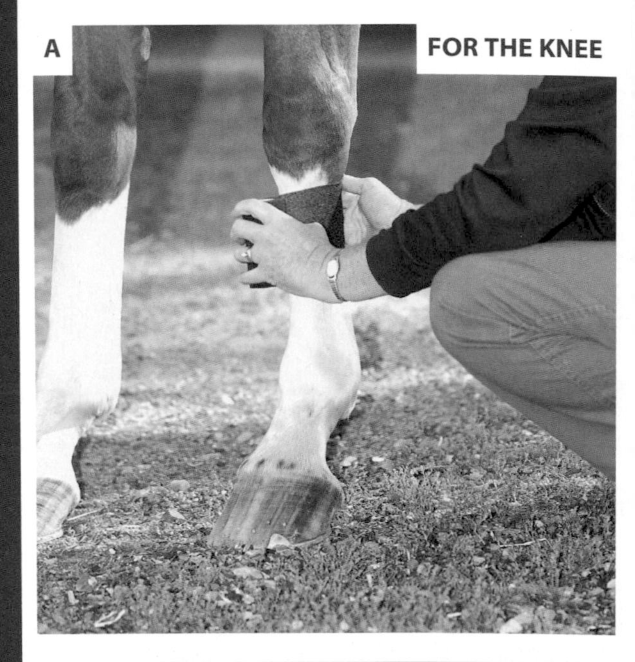

B

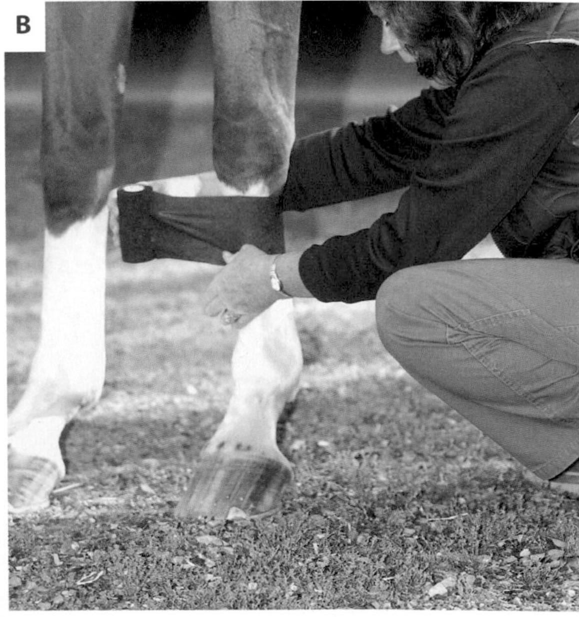

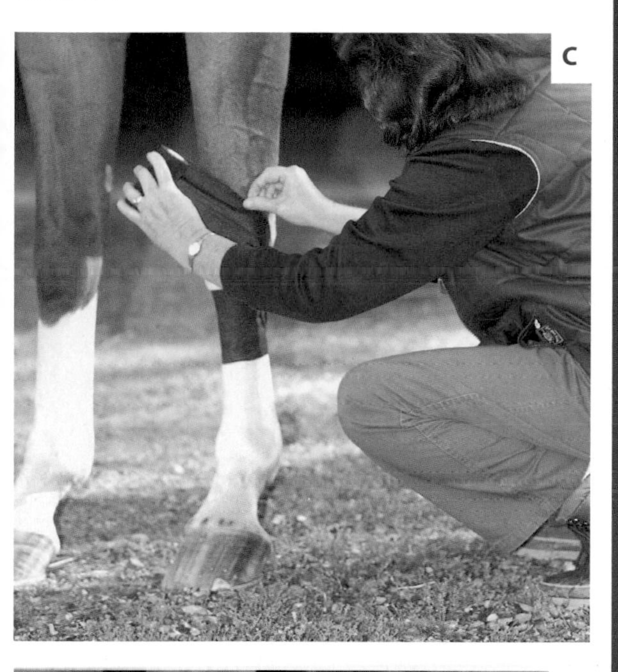
C

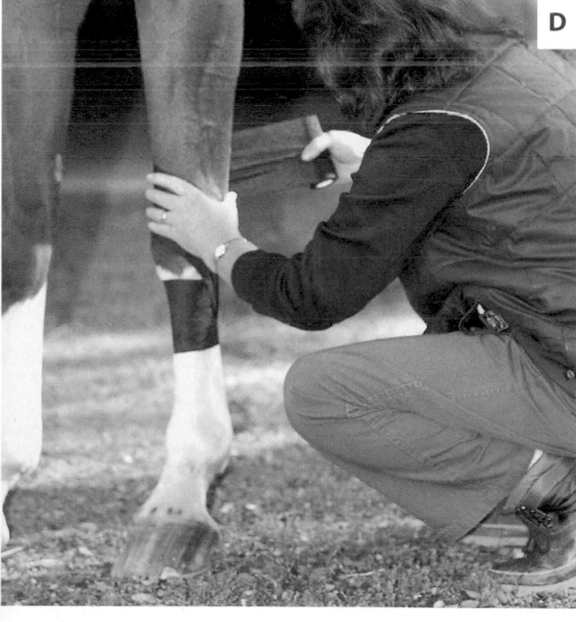
D

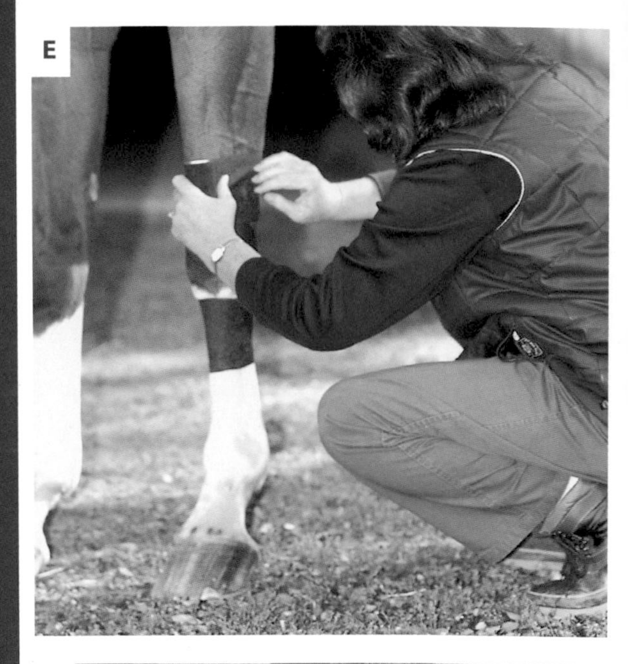
E

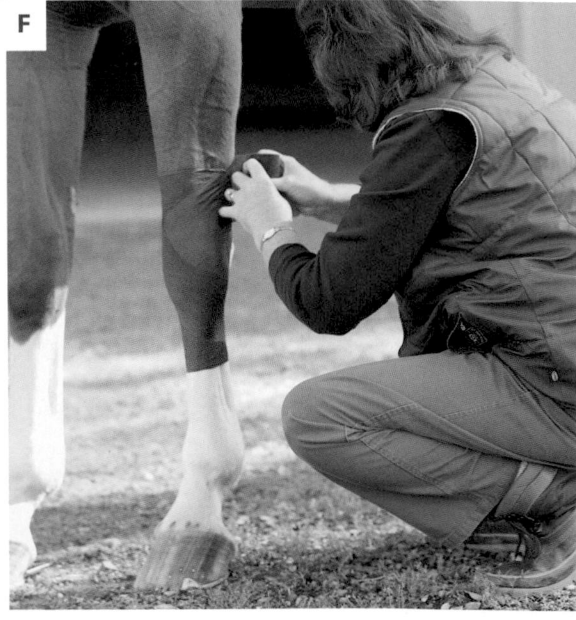
F

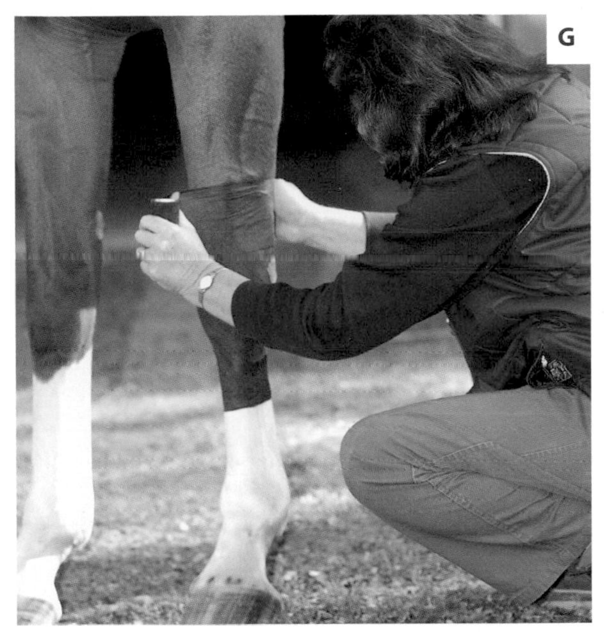
G

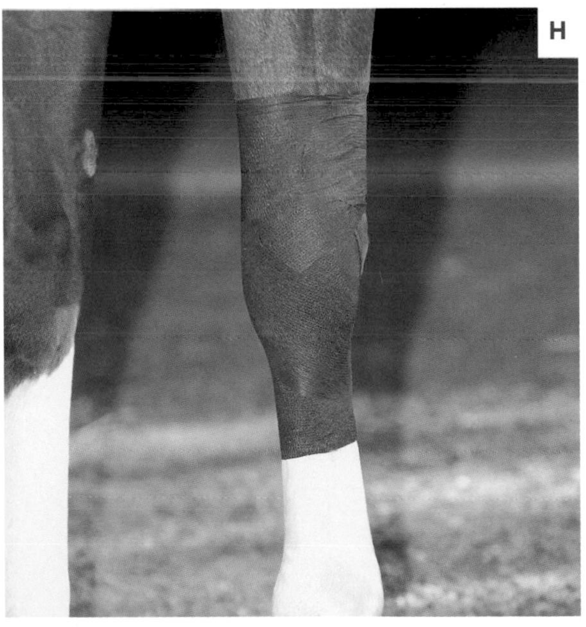
H

ADMINISTERING EYE MEDICATIONS

Eye medications can be easily given once you've had a little practice. However, it is always best to have a helper since you will need to use both hands.

- Hold the eye open by pressing on the skin above and under the limits of the eyeball with your thumb and first or second finger, pulling upward on the upper eyelid and down on the lower eyelid.
- Steady the hand holding the medication by resting it firmly against the horse's head.
- Position the tube or bottle of medication at about a 45-degree angle to the eye and 1/4 to 1/2 inch above the level of the eye.
- Keep your hand resting on the horse's head, and follow any movements he might make to avoid directly contacting and/or possibly injuring the eye. Place the medication directly onto the surface of the eye. Then allow the eyelids to close.

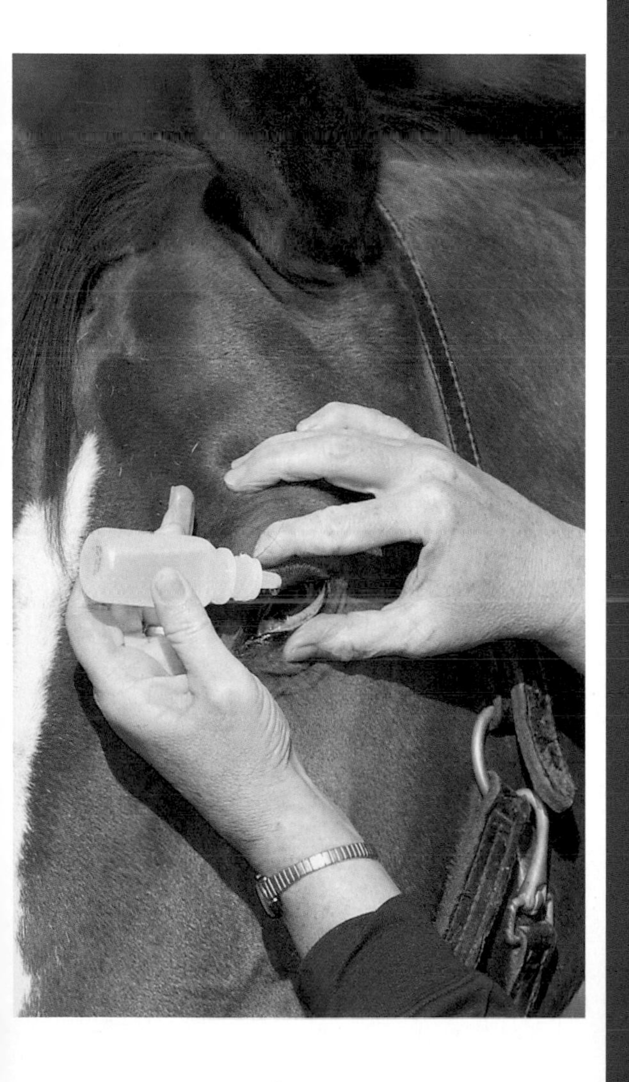

HOT VS. COLD FIRST AID THERAPY

COLD THERAPY

General rule:
Cold stops inflammation and reduces blood flow. Heat may worsen inflammation and increases blood flow.

Cold is the treatment of choice for all fresh injuries and for the first 72 hours after a new injury or flare-up of an old one. It is usually used for joint, tendon, or ligament problems but is also useful for controlling inflammation and slowing bleeding around fractures, bone bruises, hematomas, cuts/lacerations, snake bites, insect stings/bites, hives.

Cold therapy can be accomplished by soaking or hosing the affected area with cold water or by the application of iced wraps. If soaking in a tub, make sure the water is changed or ice added when the water becomes warm. Do not tub soak if the skin is broken.

Several manufacturers make icing boots specifically designed to fit horses. You can make your own cold packs by putting crushed ice into a plastic sandwich or food storage bag along with a 50:50 mixture of water and alcohol. Place this directly against the area to be cooled, and secure it with a polo wrap. Replace with a fresh wrap when the first one's ice has melted.

Cooling can be used repeatedly for the first 72 hours, or until the signs of inflammation (heat, swelling, redness) have subsided; whichever comes first. A cooling/anti-inflammatory liniment may be applied overnight or

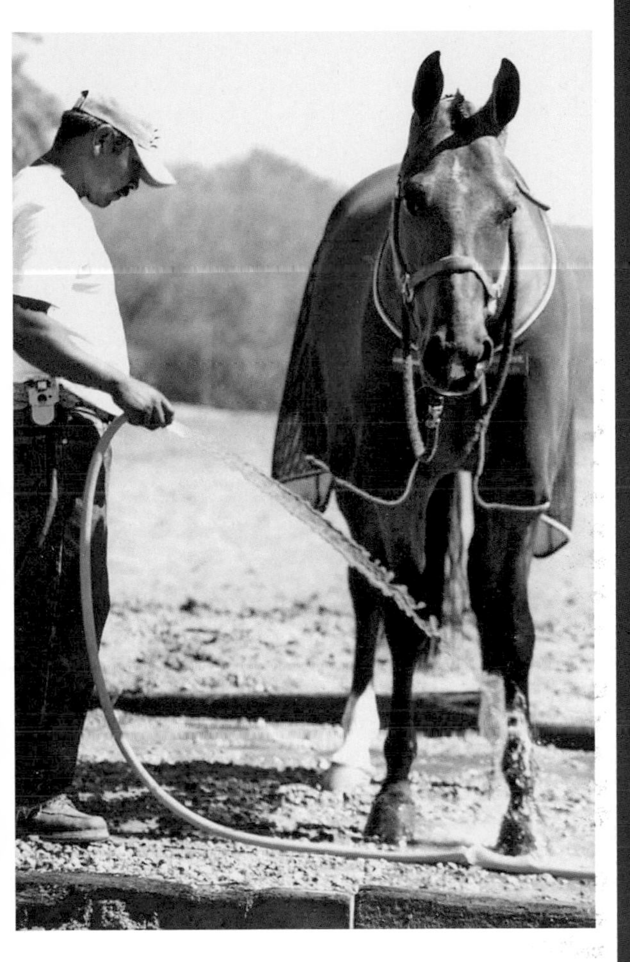

when you can't hose/ice the area. If heat and swelling persist after 72 hours, consult your veterinarian for further instructions.

CAUTIONS:

- Do not apply ice directly to skin.
- Do not apply ice packs to the horse's back or areas of muscle spasm.
- Do not use ice packs on severe burns or on

lacerations where the blood supply to the skin may not be good (check with your vet first).
- Do not use cold therapy for the feet if there is a chance the pain is caused by an abscess.

HEAT THERAPY

Therapies that heat the area and stimulate blood flow are usually not appropriate the first few days following the development of a problem because the local inflammatory response is already causing these effects. The exceptions to this are muscular spasm or strain, back pain, and abscesses. Areas can be warmed by soaking them in hot water or by applying heavy towels soaked in hot water and then covering with a layer of plastic to hold the heat (plastic trash bags or old shower curtains work well). Adding Epsom salts, 1/2 cup per gallon of water, improves the relaxing and drawing effects. Warming liniments may be used in place of hot water and in between hot water treatments.

CAUTIONS:

- Do not apply liniments without thoroughly washing off Epsom salt solution.
- Dilute liniments before use if applying right after hot soaks (pores are open).
- Discontinue liniment, or dilute it, if the horse shows pain/agitation when you apply it.
- Discontinue liniments if skin flaking or blistering develops.

PROPER USE OF LINIMENTS

A liniment, rub or gel that feels cooling on your skin may seem like the ideal thing to use on a leg that is hot and inflamed. However, a cool sensation on the skin does not mean a liniment is cooling the tissues. In fact, the end result is a mild irritant/inflammatory effect. Below is a list of typical liniment ingredients and the types of conditions where they are appropriate to use for local relief. Read the package directions to see if bandaging over the liniment is appropriate.

TYPE I, anti-inflammatory: DMSO, DMSO with steroids added, Aloe Vera, Arnica, Calendula, MSM, Artemisia (Wormwood), plain witch hazel, plain isopropyl alcohol. Use only these ingredients on acute problems.

TYPE II, warming and mildly irritant: Menthol, camphor, thymol, salicylates, Capsicum, Ruta, iodine, Echinacea, Melaleuca (tea tree). These may be used on longstanding problems or after the acute inflammation is resolved with new problems (usually about 72 hours after time of injury).

SUPPORTIVE CARE OF THE ILL OR INJURED HORSE

Good nursing care is just as important to rapid recovery as treating the specific problem or illness. Some guidelines include:

- Confine the horse in a pen, run, or large stall either alone or with one quiet buddy.
- Protect him from the weather and extremes of cold/heat by providing shelter, blankets, fans, etc.
- Arrange a comfortably bedded area for the horse to lie down.
- Provide constant access to a white salt block and fresh, clean water. Horses prefer lukewarm (about body temperature) water.
- Feed a mature cutting of grass hay, free of dust or mold, free choice or as instructed by your vet.
- Drastically reduce or eliminate grain and substitute a vitamin/mineral/protein pellet instead. Feed 2000 IU of vitamin E in oil and 4 to 6 oz. of stabilized flax seed for antioxidant nutrients. If needed, soaked beet pulp helps the horse to hold weight well while keeping him calm. Substitute beet pulp pound per pound for the grain portion of the ration if horse has trouble holding weight, or 1/2 pound (dry weight) beet pulp per pound of grain if he is overweight or gaining while confined. Mixing 8 oz. of wheat bran per pound of beet pulp, or feeding 50:50 beet pulp and plain oats, provides balanced major minerals.
- Choose a safe work place for treatments, with good footing, good lighting, high overhead clearance and room for you to maneuver.
- Understand that stressed, hurt, or sick horses usually prefer to be left alone. Work quietly and gently when doing necessary handling for hoof care, grooming, and

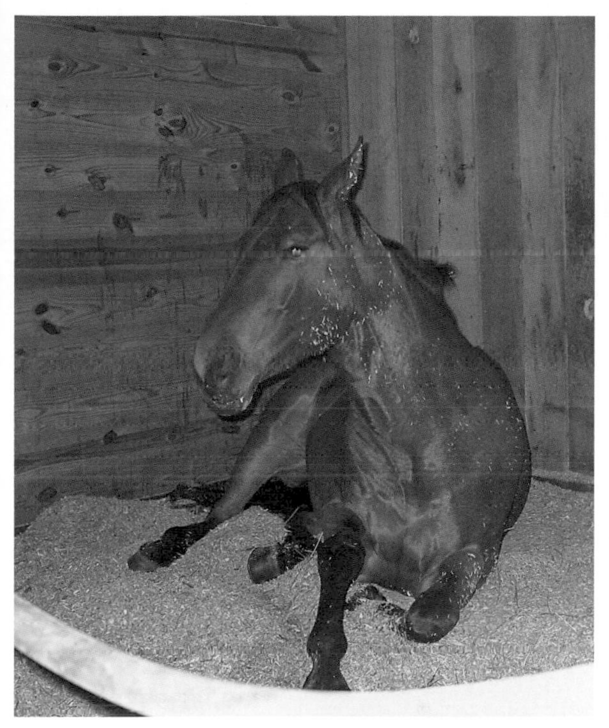

Provide the injured horse with a clean bedded area free from excess distractions.

fly control. Do not fuss over the horse unless he is obviously seeking attention.

- Be alert for changes in attitude, appetite, water consumption, urination, manure output and report these to your vet.
- Keep a notebook or clipboard near the horse and use it to record treatments, vital signs, observations regarding the problem you are treating, as well as general attitude, appetite, etc.

MAKE AN EMERGENCY ROPE HALTER

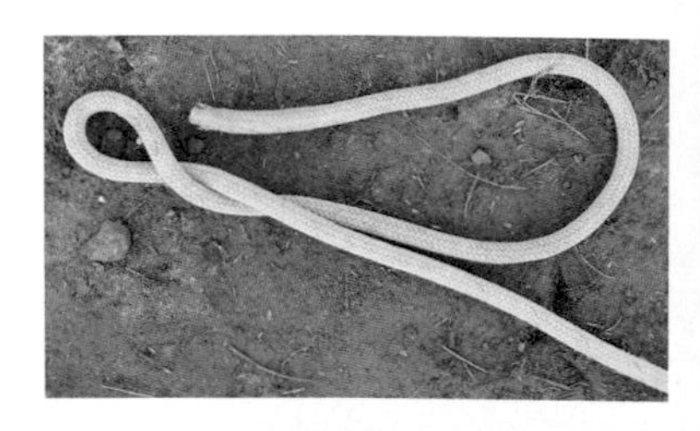

Begin with a length of rope at least 20 feet long. This emergency rope halter will fit a variety of animals — any size horse, a goat, or even a llama.

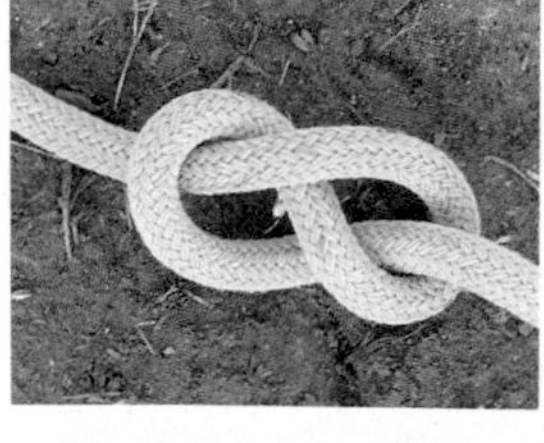

- Tie an open figure-eight knot in one end of the rope, and hold the rest looped softly in your hand. Later, you'll feed a short length of rope through the opening to complete the halter.

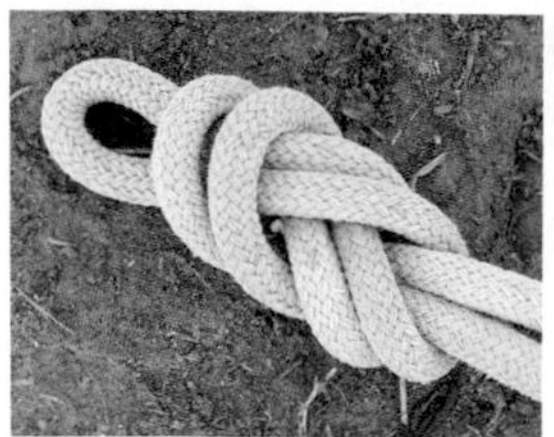

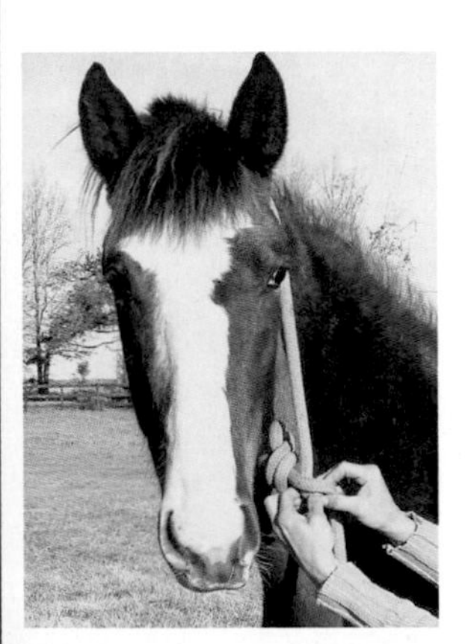

- Approach the horse from the left at the shoulder. Slip the knotted end of the rope over his neck.

- Catch the knot under his neck and gather it with the length of rope on your side, making a loop around the neck.

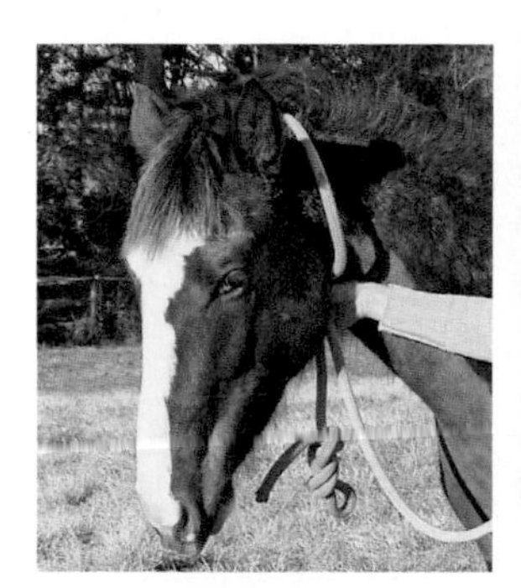

- Gently ease the rope loop up the neck toward the top of the horse's head, talking softly and keeping the horse relaxed. Do not touch the horse's ears.

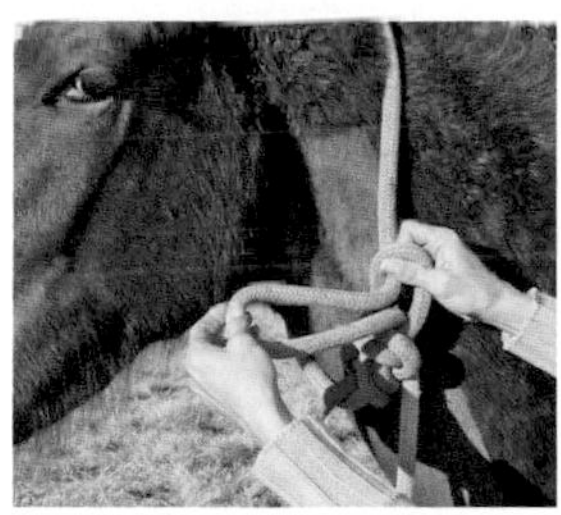

- Feed a two-foot loop of excess rope through the open knot under the horse's chin. This will become the nosepiece. Push the nosepiece up over the horse's nose.

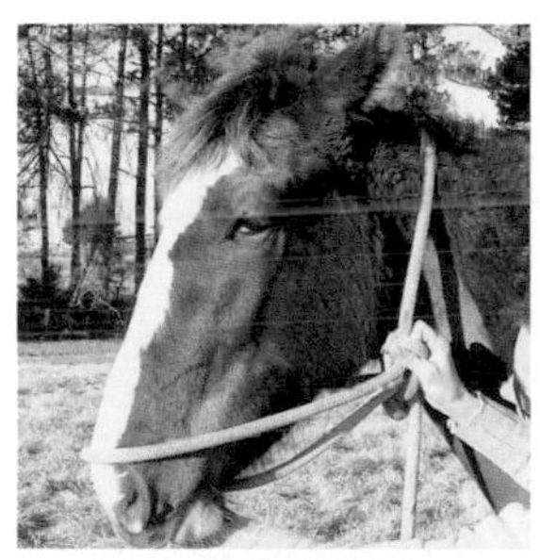

- Do not attempt to tie a horse with this halter. Hold the end of the rope but do not pull the horse by this rope, as it will tighten when pulled on or work loose and slip off the head when it isn't being held.

- Adjust the emergency halter around the nose and poll, raising it about two inches higher on the nose than you see in this photo.

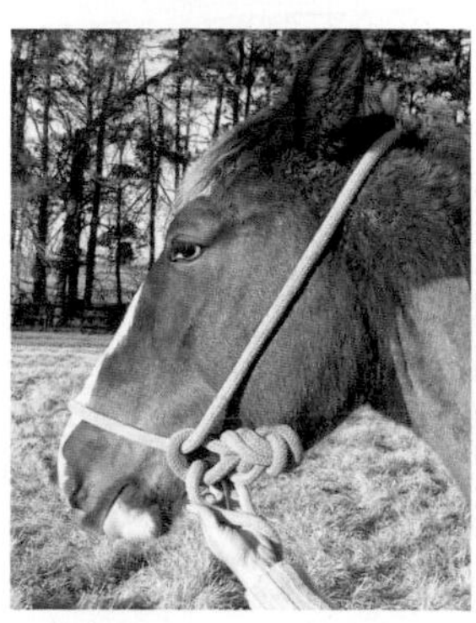

GIVING INTRAMUSCULAR INJECTIONS

The fleshy area of the horse's neck (see photo) is the most commonly used injection site, as it's the safest spot for the person doing the injection.

- Prepare the site by brushing off loose dirt and hair, washing it with soap and water and wiping it (down to skin level) with alcohol.
- Hold the needle between your thumb and first finger, touching only the hub (top).

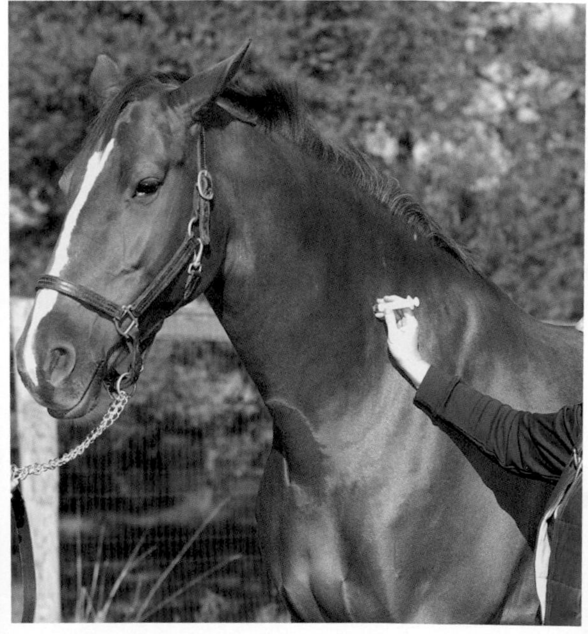

This needle is properly inserted, straight into the horse's neck muscle for its full length.

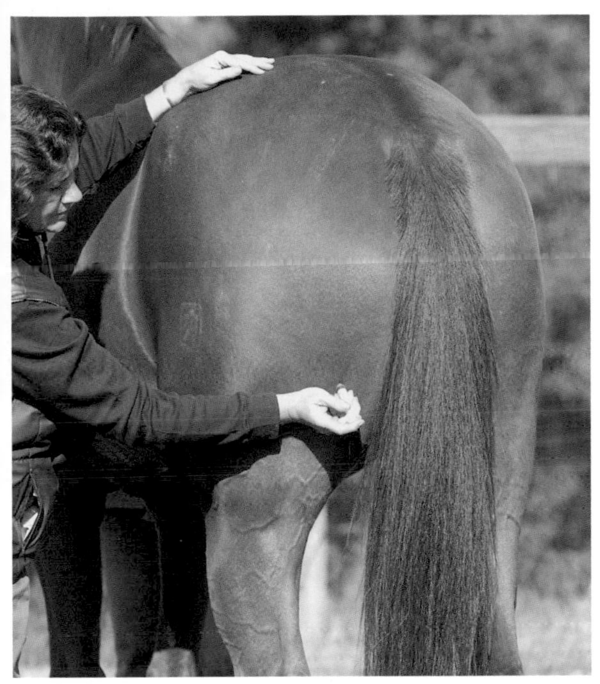

Since necks often become sore after multiple injections, alternate sites are needed. The best bet is the large muscle mass of the upper hind leg.

- Aim for the center of your target area. Quickly and forcefully place the needle deep into the muscle. This should be done in a manner similar to shooting a dart. Slow insertion, or hesitant insertion, causes much more pain. Also, do not slap or punch the horse before inserting the needle. That doesn't numb the area but does upset the horse.
- Next, securely attach the syringe containing the medication to the hub. Pull the plunger back very gently to see if the syringe fills quickly and easily with blood. If you get blood filling the syringe, remove the needle and use another spot. If you do not get blood, then inject the medication at a slow and steady pace.

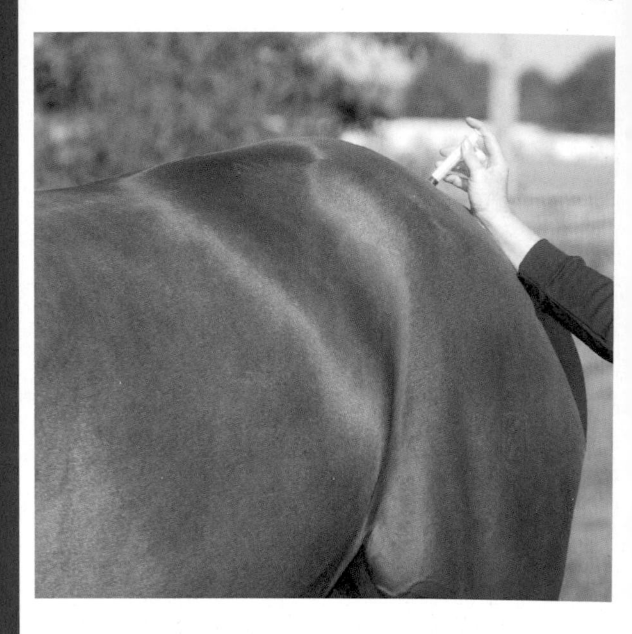

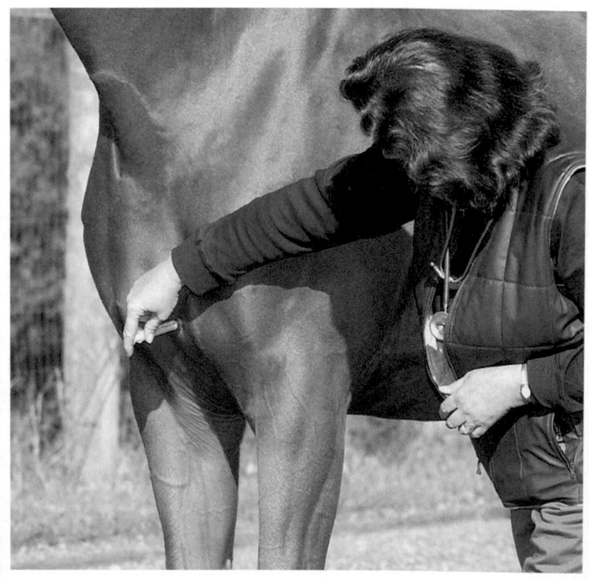

Get approval from your veterinarian before using alternative sites for intramuscular injections.

EUTHANASIA UNDER EMERGENCY CONDITIONS

As terrible as it sounds, occasionally a horse is so badly injured that the only appropriate measure is to euthanize him ("put him to sleep"). The owner is normally the only person with the legal authority to direct the euthanasia of his or her animal. In special situations or in some states, a law enforcement or animal control officer may be authorized to make this decision. If the owner is not present, or is injured or incapacitated, their agent (a person with legal permission to make decisions for the owner) may give authorization to euthanize.

Someone should explain the process of euthanasia to the horse owner and get his or her permission before acting. The owner may not want to be present during euthanasia.

Chemical euthanasia may not be available or appropriate in certain situations, in which case euthanasia by gunshot may be the only option. Whenever possible, though, you should have a veterinarian on the scene — even a small animal veterinarian, who can help with sedation prior to euthanasia. If done properly, field euthanasia with a firearm can be quick, humane, and effective.

INFORMATION FOR EMERGENCY PERSONNEL ON THE SCENE

Weapon safety

The shooter should be familiar with the safe operation and firing of guns, and take care that no one could be in the range of fire or at risk from a ricocheting bullet. The caliber of the weapon is less important than correctly placing the bullet in the brain of the animal. Even something as small as a .22 may be used. Rifles are difficult to aim properly and often have high velocity rounds that may exit the animal and heighten the risk of ricochet or bystander injury. However, if a rifle is all you have, use it extra carefully.

If the horse is in a closed area or trailer where it would be impossible to get correct aim, then the animal should be heavily sedated, given analgesics or a short-acting general anesthetic so he can be extricated from the tight spot before euthanasia.

Proper procedure for euthanasia by gunshot

Draw a line from the base of one ear to the opposite eye, and the same on the other side. Use lipstick, blood, or a marker to make sure it is correctly marked. Where the lines cross will make an X — this is the bulls-eye target for the bullet trajectory.

The muzzle of the weapon should be held at least 1/4 inch away from the skull, and at a 90-degree angle to the bone. This increases the chances of the projectile lodging in the neck and prevents ricochets.

While reflex breathing-like movements, muscular twitching, or even limb movements may occur for a few minutes after a horse has been euthanized by injection or a correctly placed bullet, be assured that the horse is dead and these reflex movements will stop quickly. The veterinarian should confirm there is no pulse or breathing before leaving the scene.

26

EQUINE FRACTURES

Emergency splinting techniques by the Center for Equine Health, UC Davis School of Veterinary Medicine

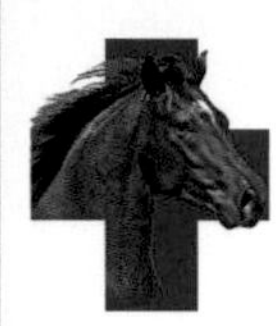

FIRST AID KIT

- Hardwood boards of varying lengths
- Plastic PVC pipe (3- and 4-inch) of varying lengths, split in half lengthwise
- Kimzey splint, if desired (availble from Kimzey Welding Works, Woodland, CA.)
- Cast padding materials such as cotton, synthetic foam or old bed pillows
- Aluminum electrical conduit
- Duct tape (2-3 rolls)
- Sterile 4x4 gauze pads/sponges (3-4 packages)
- Sterile stretchable gauze bandage (4-6 rolls)
- Medical adhesive tape (2-4 rolls)

EMERGENCY FIRST AID FOR EQUINE FRACTURE PATIENTS

1. Evaluate the patient for shock and blood loss. Keep the horse quiet and do not move it until the limb is adequately stabilized with an appropriate temporary splint.
2. Relieve pain and anxiety to achieve patient stability.
3. Clean the wound or area of injury with water. Bandage it to prevent further contamination.
4. Control blood loss by applying direct pressure over the wound with bandages. Pressure bandages should be applied before splinting is attempted
5. Stabilize the limb to prevent further trauma.

The key to stabilizing the limb is to apply an appropriate splinting device, which will prevent additional skin and muscle trauma and neurovascular disruption, and will limit damage of the fractured bone ends. The splint also provides a strut for the horse to bear a moderate amount of weight, which relieves stress and anxiety.

Correct application of splinting devices is essential because more damage can be done to the fracture if applied incorrectly. Nonetheless, not having experience in applying the appropriate splint should not be an excuse for not stabilizing the fractured limb.

EMERGENCY SPLINTING TECHNIQUES FOR STABILIZING EQUINE FRACTURES

DISTAL FORELIMB FRACTURES

Includes cannon bone, long and short pastern bones, and sesamoid bone.

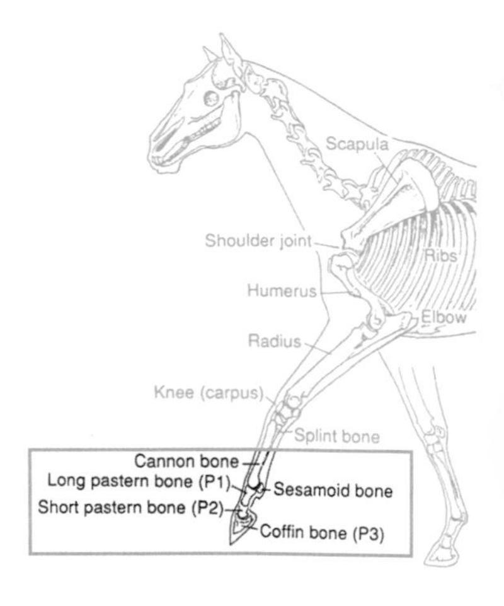

The goal of splinting is to align the bony column and protect the soft tissues in the fetlock and pastern from excessive compression. The splint should cover the entire foot and extend to the upper portion of the cannon bone. A commercially available splint that has been specifically designed for these injuries is the Kimzey Leg Saver. This splint is easy to apply and is very effective for stabilizing all of the above-listed injuries.

(Top right) The dorsal board splint must incorporate the entire foot to be effective.

(Bottom right) The Kimzey Leg Saver is easy to apply and is very effective for stabilizing lower limb fractures and suspensory apparatus failures

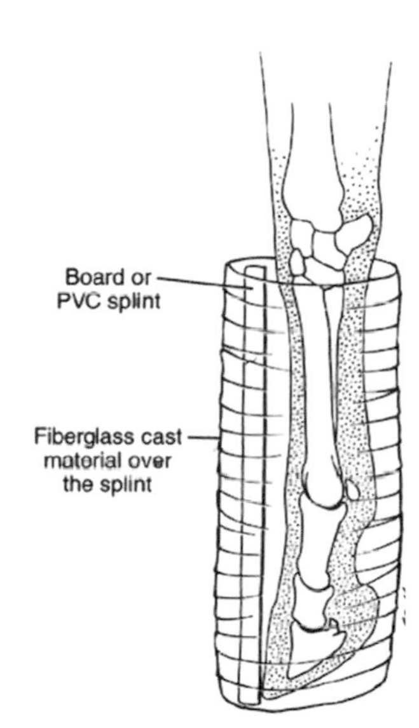

Splint Application

- Apply a bandage of medium thickness from the coronary band to the upper portion of the cannon bone.
- Place a board or other rigid material against the front lower portion of the limb and secure it with nonelastic tape or casting material. It is important to include the entire foot within the splint to avoid causing more trauma at the fracture site.
- A Kimzey Leg Saver can be applied in place of the dorsal splint.

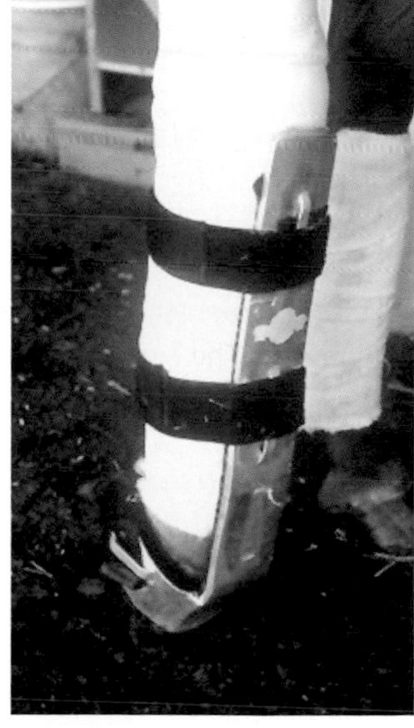

MID-FORELIMB FRACTURES

Includes cannon bone, knee, and forearm.

The goal of splinting is to realign the bony column and prevent the lower limb from moving in four directions. This is best accomplished by applying two splints placed at right angles: a caudal splint placed from the ground to the top of the olecranon (point of elbow), and a lateral splint placed from the ground to the elbow.

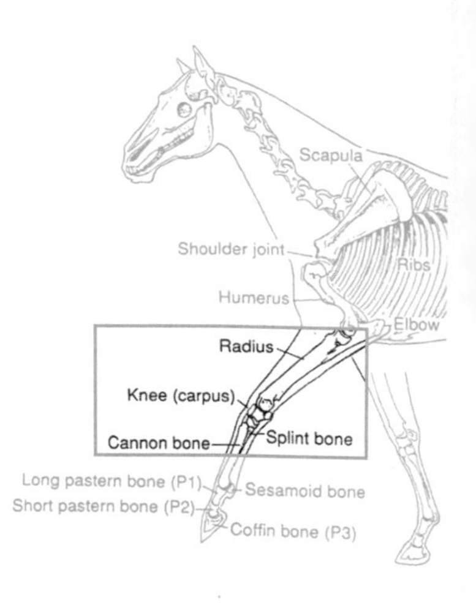

Splint Application

- Apply a bandage of moderate thickness from the coronary band to the highest point of the elbow. Typically, three levels of bandage are required to reach the elbow.
- Place a caudal splint extending from the ground to the point of elbow against the limb and secure it with nonelastic tape.
- Place a lateral splint extending from the ground to the elbow joint against the limb and secure it with nonelastic tape.
- The entire foot should be included in the splint to increase stability.

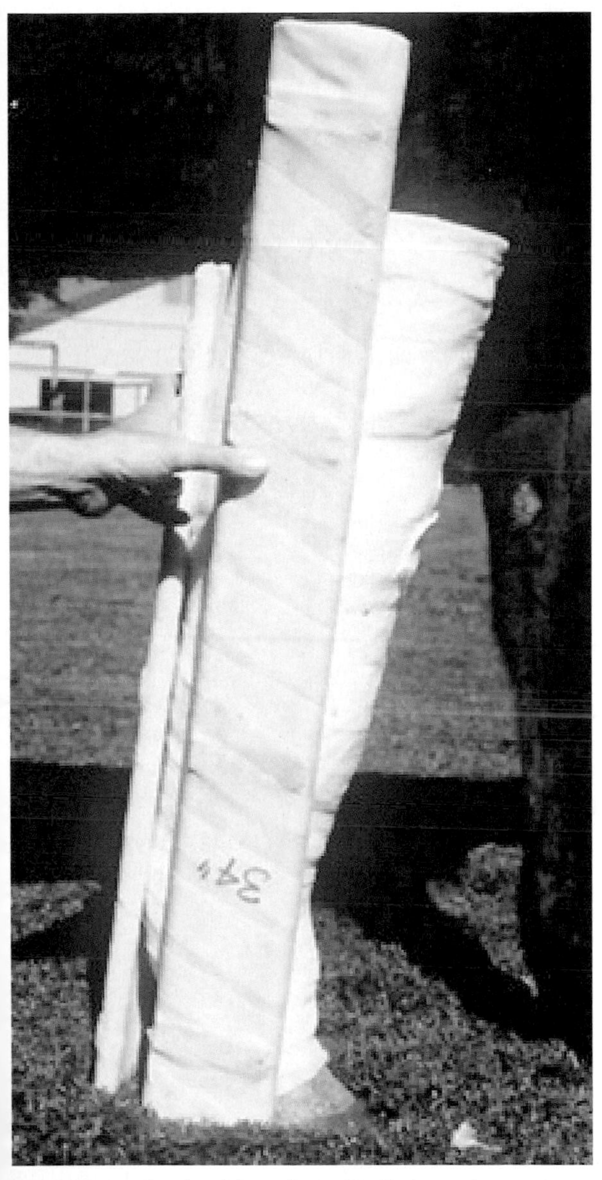

Two splints are placed at right angles to align the bony column and prevent movement.

MID-FOREARM FRACTURES

Includes the forearm above the knee.

The goal of splinting is to realign the bony column and prevent movement of the bone in any direction. Two splints should be applied at right angles: a caudal splint placed from the ground to the top of the olecranon (point of elbow), and a lateral splint placed from the ground to above the shoulder to prevent lateral movement of the limb.

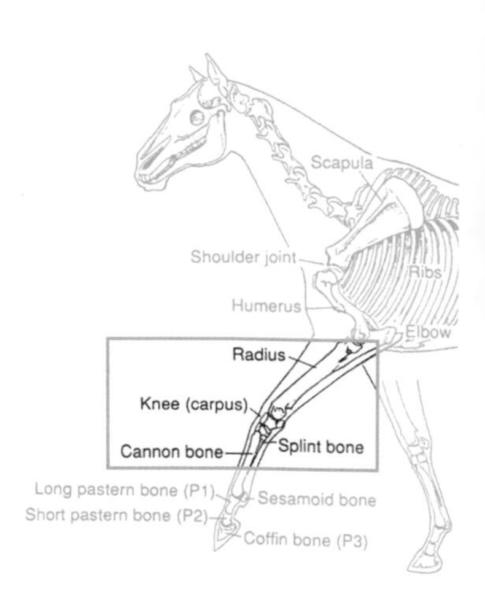

Splint Application

- Apply a bandage of moderate thickness from the coronary band to the highest point of the elbow. Typically, it will require three levels to stack the bandage to the elbow.
- Place the caudal splint from the ground to the highest point of the elbow and secure it with nonelastic tape.
- Place the lateral splint from the ground to above the shoulder joint and secure it with nonelastic tape.
- Secure the highest portion of the splint to the trunk, as shown, by wrapping elastic bandage material around the neck and chest, through the forelimbs, over the withers, and under the girth in a figure-eight pattern.

(Top right) With the lateral splint placed above the scapulohumeral joint, the lower portion of the limb cannot deviate laterally.

(Bottom right) As shown, the splint is placed to the level of the withers to ensure that it crosses the shoulder joint.

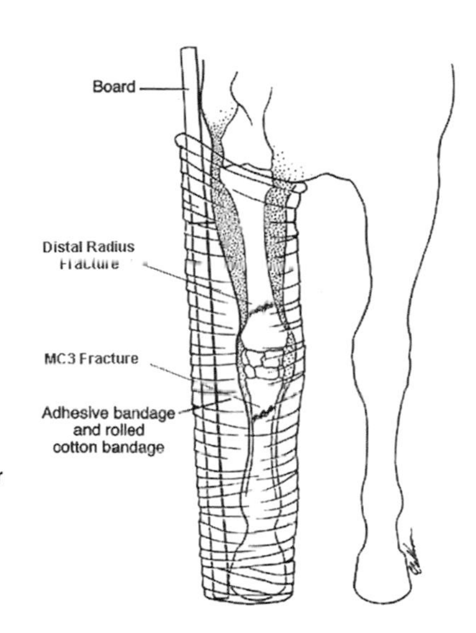

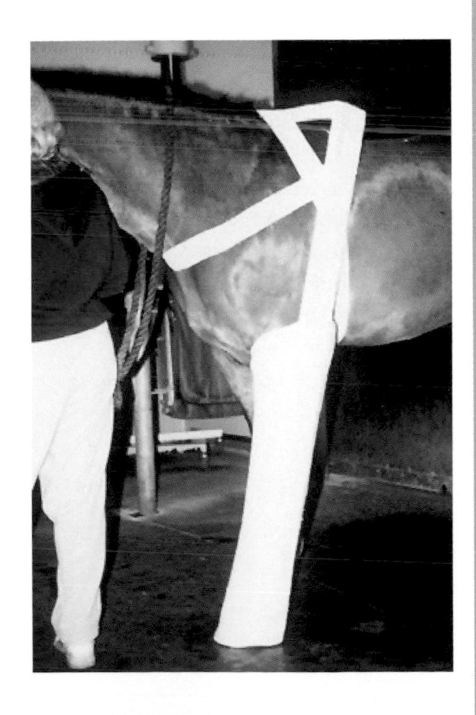

PROXIMAL FORELIMB FRACTURES

Includes the elbow, shoulder above elbow, and shoulder blade.

The goal of splinting is to fix (lock) the knee (carpus). By doing so, horses that have lost triceps function will immediately become more comfortable. Fixing the knee and aligning the bony column is best achieved by applying one splint that extends from the ground to the elbow on the caudal (rear-facing) aspect of the limb.

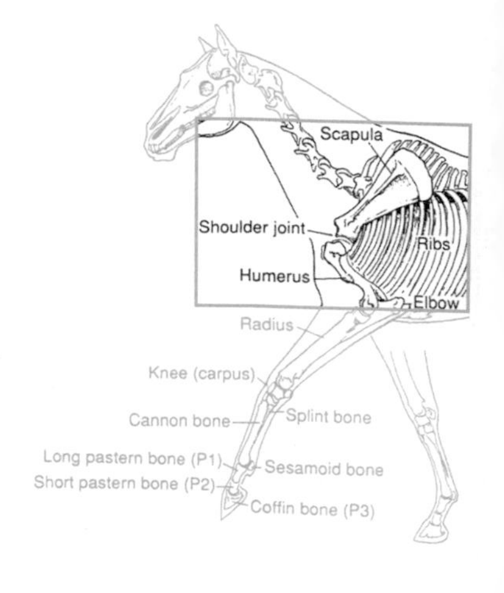

Splint Application

- Place a bandage of medium thickness from the coronary band to the highest point of the elbow. Typically it will require three levels to stack the bandage to the elbow.
- A caudal splint extending from the ground to the elbow point is taped to the limb with nonelastic tape.

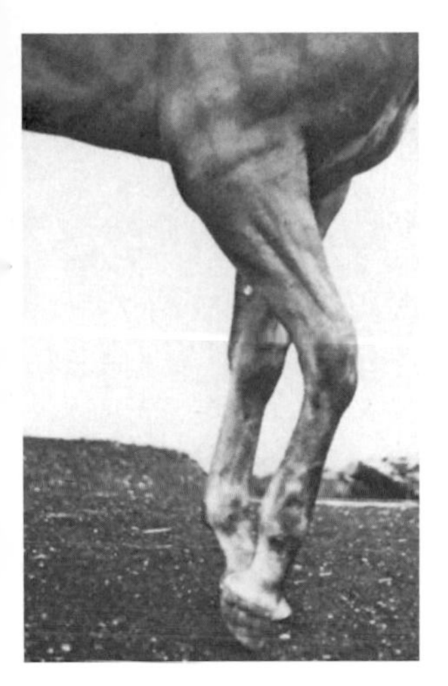

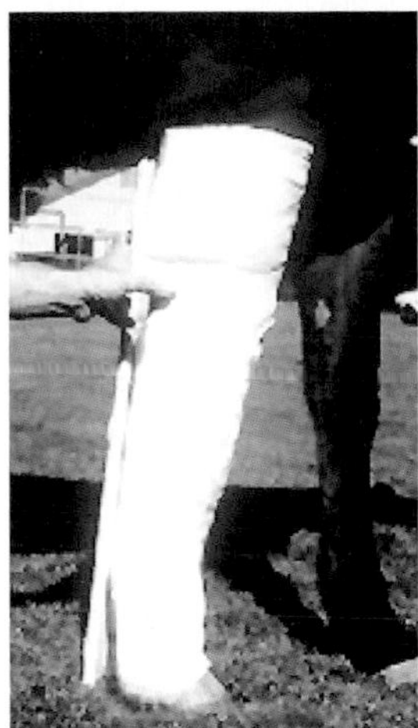

(Left) Horses that have lost triceps function cannot fix the knee and cannot bear weight on the limb.

(Right) A single splint is applied on the upper-back aspect of the limb to fix the knee and realign the bony column.

PROXIMAL LIMB FRACTURES

Includes shoulder blade.

Splinting is contraindicated, either above or below the fracture, and could increase trauma directly at the fracture site.

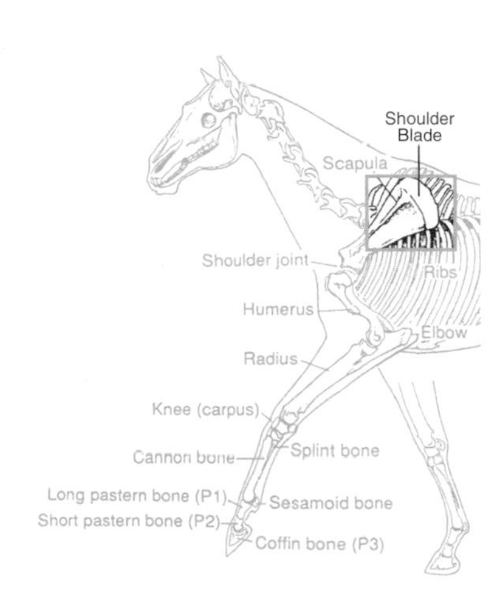

DISTAL HINDLIMB FRACTURES

Includes lower cannon bone, sesamoid bone, and long and short pastern bones.

The goal of splinting, as with the forelimb, is to align the bony column and protect the soft tissues in the fetlock and pastern from excessive compression. This can best be accomplished by applying a splint on the plantar (lower-back) aspect of the limb. The splint should incorporate the entire foot and extend to the highest portion of the cannon bone. The Kimzey splint is very effective for these fractures.

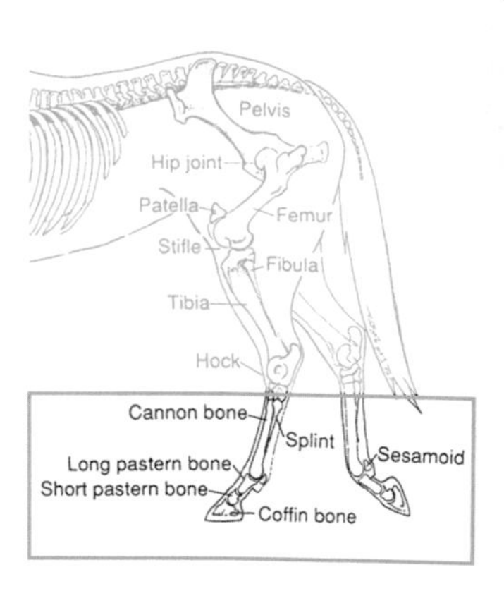

Splint Application

- Apply a bandage of medium thickness from the coronary band to the top of the cannon bone.
- Place a board or other rigid material at the lower-back aspect of the limb and secure it with nonelastic tape. It is very important to incorporate the entire foot within the splint to have it be effective. If the entire foot is not incorporated, it will cause more trauma at the fracture site.
- A Kimzey Leg Saver is as effective as a plantar splint.

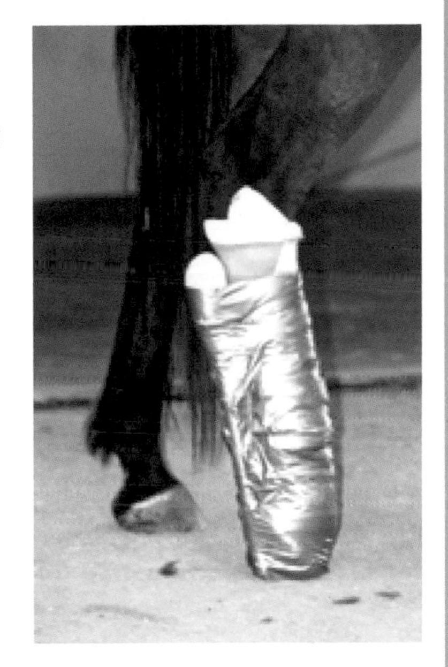

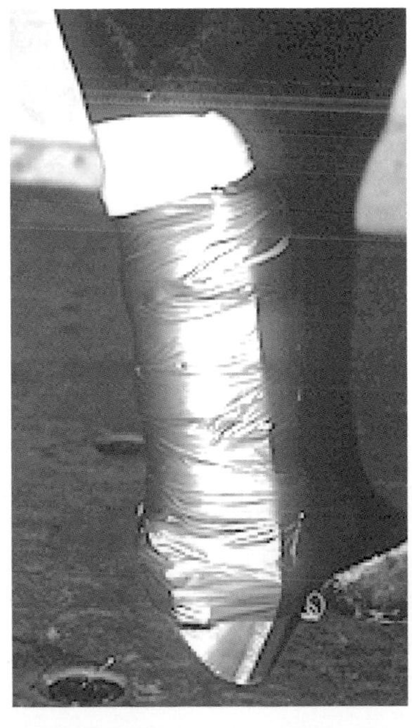

(Top) A plantar splint is placed to realign the bony column and protect the plantar soft tissues. (Bottom) A Kimzey splint is easy to apply and is very effective for stabilizing these fractures.

MID-HINDLIMB FRACTURES

Includes cannon bone and hock.

The goal of splinting is to realign the bony column and prevent movement in any of the four directions (back, front and sides). This is best accomplished by applying two splints placed at right angles: a caudal splint placed from the ground to the highest point of the hock, and a lateral splint placed from the ground to the hock. For fractures involving the tarsal bones, the lateral splint should be bent in the shape of the hindlimb to extend the splinting device higher up.

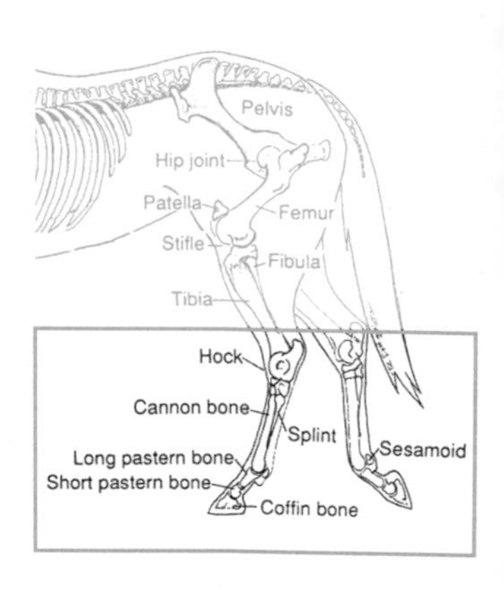

Splint Application

- Apply a bandage of moderate thickness from the coronary band to the stifle (see skeleton). Typically, three levels of bandage are required to reach the appropriate level.
- Place a caudal splint extending from the ground to the highest point of the hock against the limb and secure it with nonelastic tape.
- Place a lateral splint extending from the ground to the highest point of the hock, or to the stifle (as in photograph), against the limb and secure it with nonelastic tape.
- The entire foot should be included in the splint.

(Top right) A lateral and caudal splint, placed to the highest point of the hock, can stabilize these fractures.

(Bottom right) A lateral splint, bent in the shape of the limb, should be used for tarsal bone fractures and dislocations or simply for greater stability.

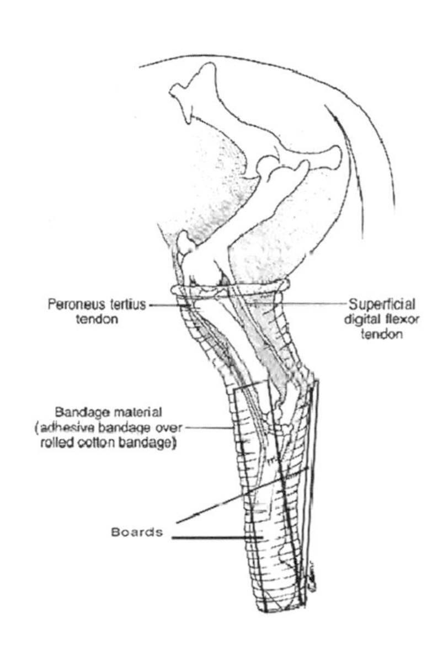

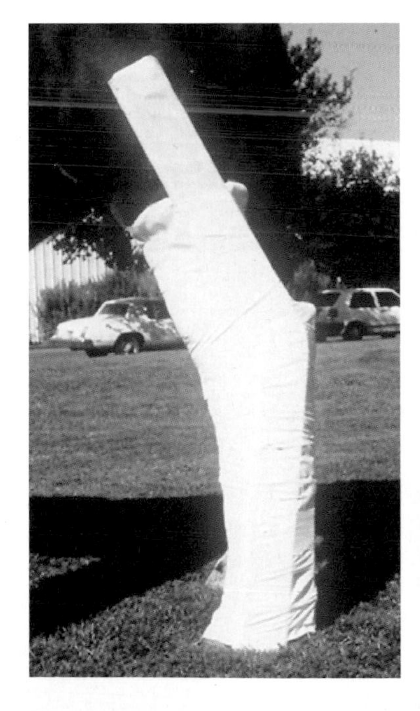

MID-PROXIMAL HINDLIMB FRACTURES

Includes hock, tibia, fibula, and stifle (gaskin area).

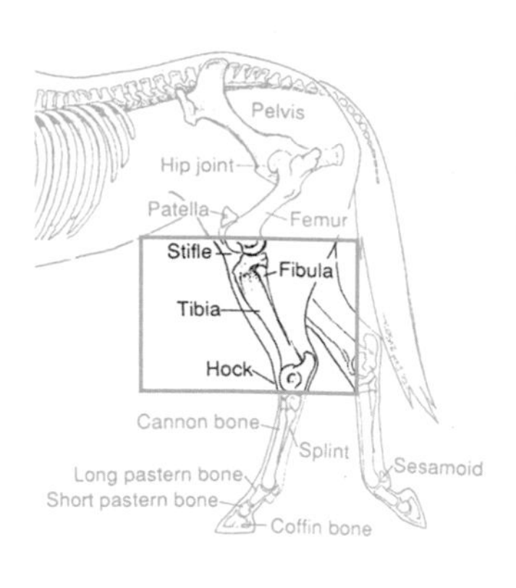

Sharp bone ends from these fractures can traumatize skin, muscle, and surrounding neurovascular structures every time the limb is flexed or extended. The goal of splinting is to realign the bony column and prevent fracture collapse as well as movement of the limb. This is best accomplished by applying one lateral splint extending from the ground to the hip. A caudal splint is contraindicated.

Splint Application

- Apply a bandage of moderate thickness from the coronary band to the stifle. Typically, three levels of bandage are required to reach the appropriate level.
- Place a lateral splint extending from the ground to the hip against the limb and secure it with nonelastic tape.
- Secure the upper portion of the splint with elastic tape placed over the hip, through the legs, under the flank, and over the lumbar spine in a figure-eight pattern.
- It is important to incorporate the entire foot in the splint.

(Top right) A lateral splint placed from the ground to the hip will effectively stabilize complete tibial fractures.

(Bottom right) The upper portion of the lateral splint is secured with elastic tape placed over the hip in a figure-eight pattern.

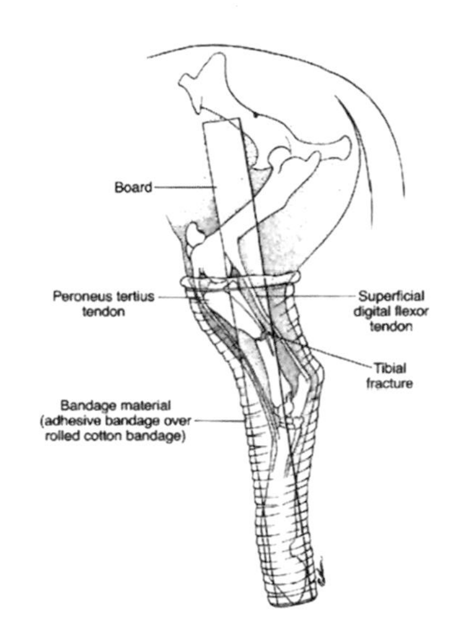

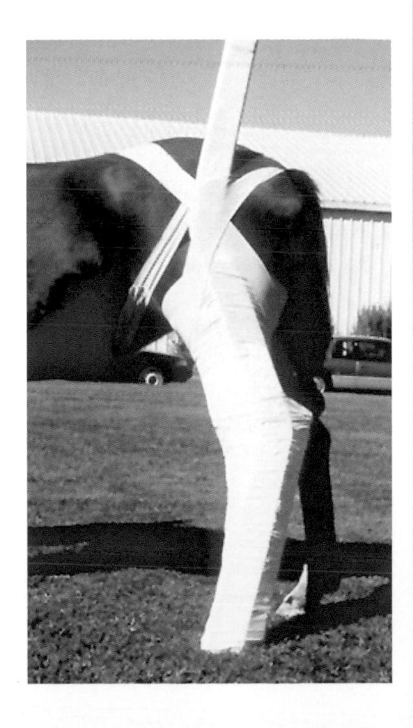

MID-PROXIMAL HINDLIMB FRACTURES

Includes the femur between the stifle and the hip joint and the pelvis.

Splinting for fractures located above the stifle is contraindicated and could increase trauma directly at the fracture site.

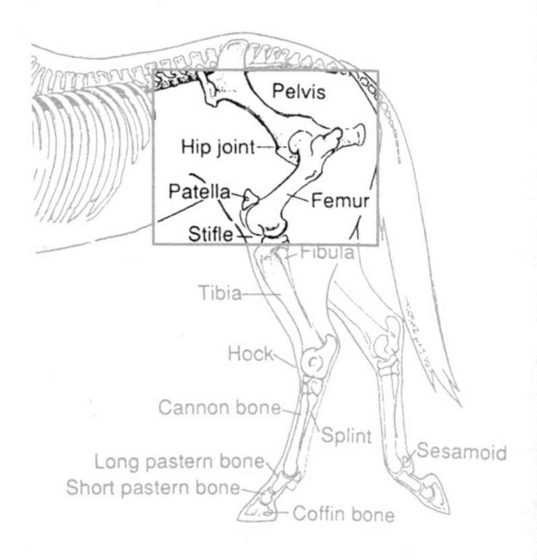

27

TRAILER ACCIDENTS & TRAPPED HORSES

Advice from Dr. Rebecca Gimenez, primary instructor, Technical Large Animal Emergency Rescue (TLAER).

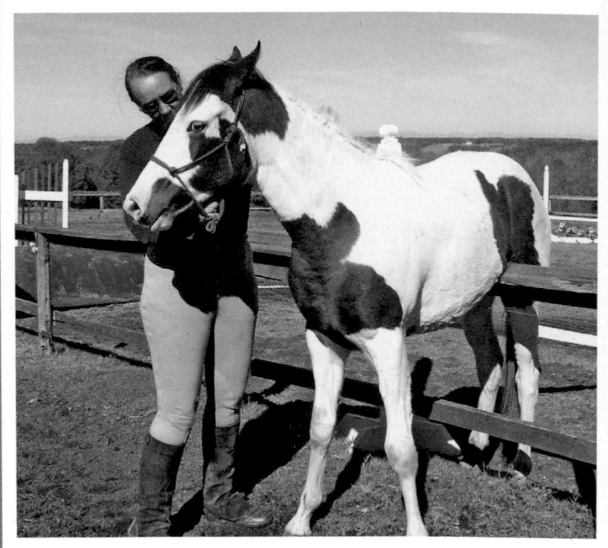

Horses can get themselves into all kinds of predicaments. This owner is staying by the horse's head to calm him, lest he do more damage trying to free himself. Someone has gone for help to cut the arena fence.

TRAILER ACCIDENTS AND TRAPPED HORSES

The best thing to do in an accident or horse-related emergency is to stay calm — the person who knows the most about an individual horse may be you. The situations discussed in this book are true emergencies where people can be seriously injured. Never attempt to assist a horse alone. In rescue situations, a terrified horse — even the family pet that would never intentionally hurt anyone — may be extremely strong and dangerous. Get professional help from the beginning.

Do not expose yourself or another person to injury or possible death while trying to save an animal. There are many documented situations where people have been seriously injured trying to assist a trapped or injured animal. Wait for professional rescue personnel if a horse is trapped. Encourage bystanders to stay quiet and disturb the horse as little as possible while the team makes a plan to extricate the animal.

CALL FOR HELP

Call a veterinarian immediately. Consider calling emergency responders (fire, police, EMS, park ranger, animal control) who will have extrication knowledge and special cutting tools. Local fire/rescue departments may not have training in the technical aspects of animal rescue, but with veterinary supervision using the resources they already have, they can apply their knowledge of human rescue to a 1,200-pound frightened animal.

One common mistake is that people fail to organize the rescue prior to beginning it. They may call friends and neighbors in and spend a lot of time trying this and that, exhausting themselves and the trapped horse. Instead, they should call for professional help, and make a careful assessment of the situation.

The vet may consider anesthesia or sedation depending on the medical stability of the animal — generally you should allow them to use their expertise and not administer any drugs you might have on hand without the veterinarian's approval. In rescue situations, drugs can actually lessen a horse's chance of survival. If you get prior authorization from the vet over the phone to drug the horse, remind the vet upon arrival that the horse has been drugged.

HANDLING THE HORSE

Ideally, the horse will be wearing a halter. Be sure whatever lead rope you use is reliable. The halter and lead are for guidance and control, however, do not let anyone yank the horse out by the halter. In general, do not use the head, neck, or legs for anchors to pull an animal out of entrapment — use the larger surface area and skeletal support of the body with webbing to reduce injury and increase success. (Think of it this way: A human victim would not be extricated from a car by placing a rope around his or her neck.) A review of actual rescues has revealed that although many animals survived the rescue, the prognosis for a good recovery was greatly reduced by injuries to the soft tissues of the lower legs, head, and neck received during the rescue.

If you have no other option than a rope and halter, increase the surface area against the skin by protecting under the halter or rope with some type of padding (t-shirt, towel, shipping boot, etc.)

Blindfolds do calm some horses, but in rare instances, the horse may become more frantic. If a blindfold (shirt, towel, cloth) is used, it should be loose on the horse's head so that if he gets up and runs off, it will fall off. Loose, blindfolded animals run in a straight line until they hit something.

Horses do not like to lie in lateral recumbency (on their sides), but prefer to be resting on their chest and stomach. Even if the horse can't get up on his own, he'll try to get onto his chest. If a horse has been on his side, you can expect that, as he's being lifted or moved he'll begin leg and neck movements in an effort to rise and stabilize himself. Use caution and stay clear of his legs. Keep a head rope on the horse and someone on the other end of it that knows what they're doing.

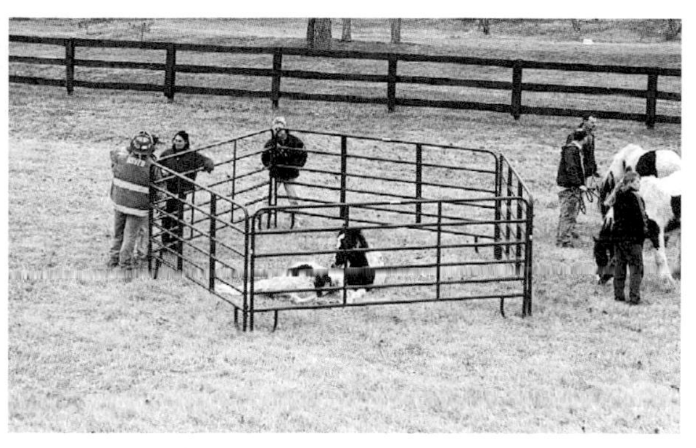

Portable pens or an existing round pen or small paddock can be useful for protecting and confining animals that are injured in disasters such as barn fires.

Never pull a horse by a rope on the halter, or by the halter itself (risk of neck/spinal cord injury). If leg ropes must be used, pad the area under the rope with cloth (a shirt, leg wrap, etc.). Instruct personnel never to fight a horse that is resisting the pull of the rope — i.e., don't pull back. If the horse resists, stop pulling and wait for him to stop pulling.

If the horse is panicked and thrashing/struggling, but extrication is not imminent, try to get some padding in the trailer in the area of the head. Horses can do serious damage to their heads.

AFTER THE RESCUE

Just because the horse is standing and grazing after being rescued, does not mean that he is okay. This is where veterinary evaluation and treatment may be most crucial — what looks like a tiny scratch to you might become a punctured septic joint in a few days, or the horse could have internal injuries. Hose (warm water and towel dry) clean the animal so that the veterinarian can see any possible injuries. In some situations, the animal may be too cold and fragile for hosing, so remove excess mud gently by hand.

After thoroughly examining the horse, the vet may prescribe pain relief or anti-inflammatory medications. Fluid therapy may be required, because stressed horses become dehydrated quickly. Anti-inflammatory and pain-killing medications, such as Banamine or phenylbutazone should only be used under veterinary supervision. If the horse was down for a long time, there may be skin damage along pressure points, such as the hips.

Shock may not be apparent until after the rescue, so watch the horse carefully for depression and weakness developing over the next few hours. Record the horse's temperature twice daily for a week after the rescue and check for any visible evidence of developing infections, like swelling or pain.

ON THE ACCIDENT SCENE
Advice to Rescue Personnel

In many cases, human rescue techniques can be used with horses, keeping in mind that a frightened, large animal can be dangerous. The same ideas of primary triage and giving first aid can apply. Be especially careful to afford the horses the same support during the extrication, and packaging for transport to definitive care that you would for a person – don't pull the horse by his head, neck, tail or legs.

Veterinary support is crucial to the success and safety of the scene. Horse people on the scene should be used as part of the incident operations team to help keep

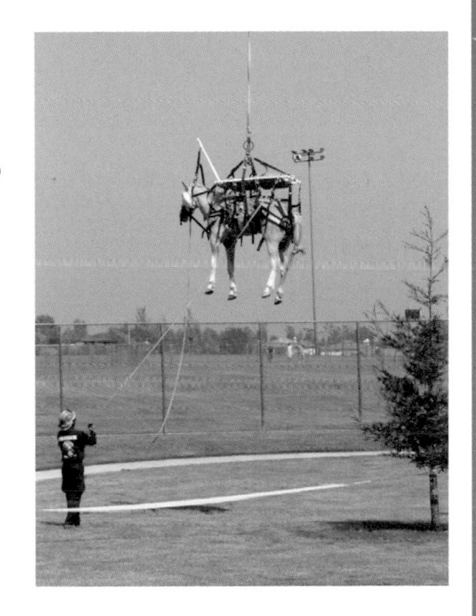

Large Animal Technical Rescue Teams practice with a trained and tranquilized horse so they're able to achieve these extraordinary rescues safely.

emergency responders safe around the animal. Horses have a strong flight instinct and are easily panicked.

- Turn off sirens once on the scene. Leave on whatever on strobes, lights and warning flashers are necessary for safety.
- Set up scene security to prevent owners from getting into an unsafe position in an attempt to help their horse, i.e., rushing into a burning barn.
- While the owner may be distraught, they may be the only "horse person" on the scene and can be invaluable in keeping the horse calm. Explain that they have a vital role to play in the rescue in this respect and need to keep their emotions under control.
- When the rescue requires moving the horse, use forward assist or backwards drag, making sure to use webbing around the horse's torso, rather than rope around his head, neck or legs. Don't use winches to extricate animals. Instead use rope systems (padded) or human power on rope.

WHEN THE HORSE CANNOT STAND

- Do not try to make the horse get up — it will excite and exhaust the horse and may worsen or cause injuries.
- If the animal is injuring itself struggling to get up, someone can put pressure on the neck and hold the head down with a blindfold. Groom, stroke, and soothe with calm voice.
- If the horse is laterally recumbent (flat on his side), try to roll horse over to relieve pressure on organs and prevent pressure sores. It's best to get the horse into sternal recumbency (up on chest) with hay bales, etc., to stabilize him.
- Roll or lay horse onto a gate with a board attached on top to move him in out of weather, alternately roll the horse onto a tarp to pull him to a shelter.
- Get temperature, pulse, and respiration (TPR) to report to the veterinarian, and provide first aid. Do not give any drugs to a downed horse unless advised by a veterinarian.
- If the horse is not on his side, offer him hay or grass and water.

TO LIFT A RECUMBENT HORSE

A simple vertical-lift system using webbing around the horse and padded ropes to a dual overhead lift system is effective to lift a horse for a short-term (15 minutes) lift. However, the horse must be able to stand after the lift, if not, more elaborate long-term sling systems should be used (Anderson Sling, Liftex Sling). These professional sling systems have been used to keep horses off their feet for months at a time; however, they require 24-hour nursing care. Try to use lower-tech, less dangerous methods whenever possible.

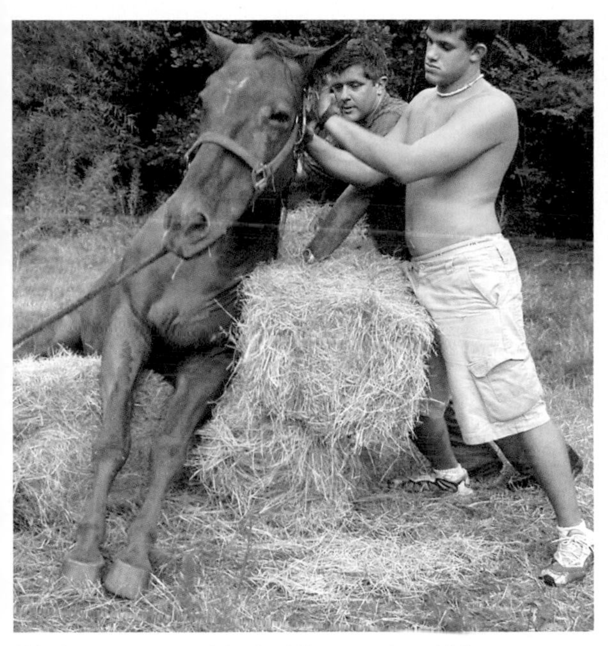

If the horse cannot stand, he should be propped up with hay or straw bales so he can be on his sternum, rather than on his side for a prolonged period.

- Get a veterinarian on scene to provide first aid and to sedate the horse if necessary, especially if a cutting tool will be used. Plug the horse's ears and protect his eyes, if possible.
- Be aware that trapped animals will frequently realize they're trapped and lie still. However, as soon as they feel a release, they may try to flee explosively, even if they're not fully free.
- In the case of a trailer accident, stabilize the trailer and separate the vehicle from the trailer, if it makes sense to do so. Coordinate for alternate trailer transport once the animals are freed.
- With a horse that cannot stand, consider transport on a board strapped to a gate, a heavy tarp folded up

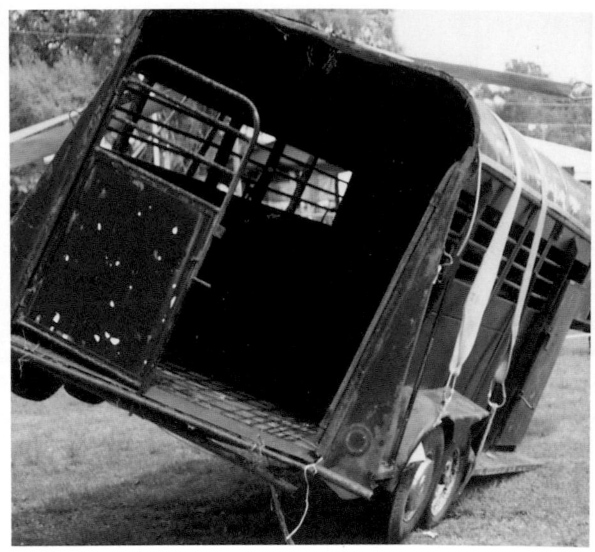

Righting a tipped trailer is the best option for sliding the animals out after all obstacles have been removed. This requires webbing around both sides of the trailer to the axles, which cradles the trailer for a slow and safe manipulation.

around the horse, or on a Rescue Glide or a simple vertical web lift, where appropriate. In many cases, sedation will be required, as the horse is likely to struggle when moving begins.

EMERGENCY SITUATIONS: Plan of action

Horse trailer accident

- Turn on warning flashers. Apply the parking brake and turn the vehicle off.
- Have someone call 911 and give them particulars on the accident.

- Have someone call a large animal veterinarian in the local area.
- Stay out of traffic lanes. Have someone set out warning triangles and flares.
- If there is a person in the trailer — either the living quarters or the horse area, check on them first.
- If horses are loose on roadway, contain them, or have a person hold them with a halter and lead rope. Do not tie them to anything. (If a semi or fire truck comes along they will break free.)
- Have someone call for another transport and stabling for the animals if trailer is not able to be hauled.
- Check on the horses through a window or opening (**do not** let anyone open a door or go into the trailer as that stimulation is likely to cause the horse to struggle).
- If you can do so safely, check to be sure that a horse has not fallen and his being held up/hung up by the tie or cross ties. If this is the case, release the horse's head immediately.
- When the horse seems quiet, if you can get into the trailer to get to the horse's head without being in danger of being struck by the legs, do so and calm the horse. When possible to do so without putting yourself in danger, remove all fallen equipment from the area of the horse so that rescue personnel have access to him.
- If you can safely do so, move the trailer out of the traffic lanes. If the trailer is still on its wheels, chock the wheels with a block of wood, a rock, or whatever you can find.
- Assess the health of the horse(s) through the window (watch nostril flare, assess general attitude, etc.).
- Do not let the horses out of the trailer without halters and lead ropes to restrain them. It's best not to let the horses out of the trailer until you have help — they may get loose and cause a secondary accident.
- Try to remove tack, obstacles, rubber mats to make a clear path to the horses for rescuers, unless your moving around will cause the horse to get restless.

- Do not attempt to put the trailer on its side, unless absolutely necessary, as horses will fight being in this position.
- Once help has arrived, give first aid for injuries, and treat the horse for heat or cold exposure.

Horse fallen through trailer floor

- Stop immediately on roadside when you hear anything unusual — put on flashers and check the horses. If a horse's leg is through the trailer floor, call Fire/Rescue/EMS and a veterinarian immediately.
- If the animal is injuring itself struggling, try a blindfold. If the vet advises and you have veterinary drugs for sedation on hand, give the correct dosage for weight.
- If possible without further upsetting or injuring the downed horse, remove any other horses from the trailer.
- Stay as close to the horse's head as you safely can, calming him until help arrives.

Horse in swimming pool or steep-sided canal

- Attempt to get the animal to shallow water to stand, or swim it to a nearby beach. Allow animal to walk out up the steps, if it will.
- Attempt to get a halter and long rope on animal's head for guidance. Don't pull the animal out by the head.
- Recognize there may be significant danger to anyone entering the water with the animal. See if you can lead the horse from a boat, though that carries dangers of its own, such as if the horse pulls or the boat capsizes.
- Don't try to make a ramp for the horse out of plywood, hay or ladders.
- Drain pool if feasible, or pump it to where water level is lower. This gives the team more time to make a decision on the type of rescue to attempt.
- Provide inflated inner-tube around the horse's neck or under his chin, for floatation.

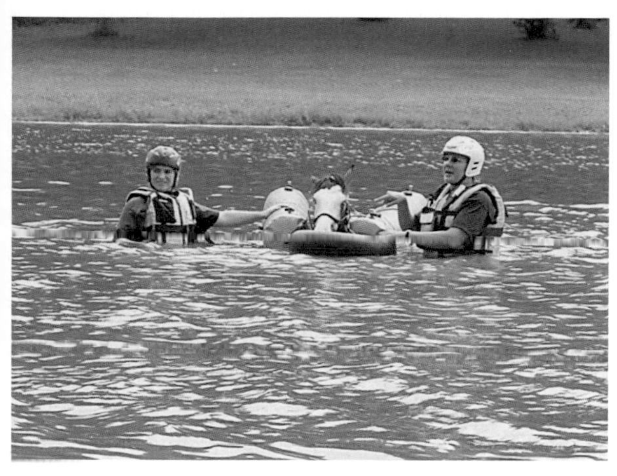

This tired horse has had flotation devices put around him to prevent him from drowning. Pieces of inflated fire hose work well also if tied beside the horse, not under it. His chin should rest on a inflated inner tube.

- If the horse has fallen through a pool cover, cut the cover from around the horse, unless it is providing floatation.
- Do not sedate the horse unless the horse is secured in a lift and struggling against it.
- Give hay or grass to calm the animal if the horse is able to stand (not having to swim), and only if the horse is already fairly calm.
- Use a forward assist (webbing around torso) to pull the animal out.
- The lasso-and-pull method is not recommended except in extreme cases where the animal is drowning anyway.
- Consider simple vertical web lift of animal.
- Don't drag the horse across a concrete edge, use a tarp to protect his skin.

Horse in ditch, ravine, mud, septic tank

- Make sure the horse can breathe, and use floatation to keep his nose above water or mud.
- Do what you can, depending upon the position of horse, but do not get between his legs or where the horse could struggle and fall on someone. Don't let humans get stuck in mud or go into a septic tank unprotected. Don't let people into a trench situation without shoring.
- Determine if a simple trail can be cut out of the ravine to walk the horse out. Considering the horse's ability to move, determine if a ramp can be built or if you can remove a wall. Remove obstacles to make a clear path around animal and in the direction of movement. Dig wall of dirt away, then roll horse to allow his feet under him and he may get up.
- Call a sump pump company or septic tank service to drain the septic tank.
- Determine if rescue professionals can inject air or water into mud around horse to negate the vacuum effect of the mud, which may be equivalent to twice the weight of the animal.

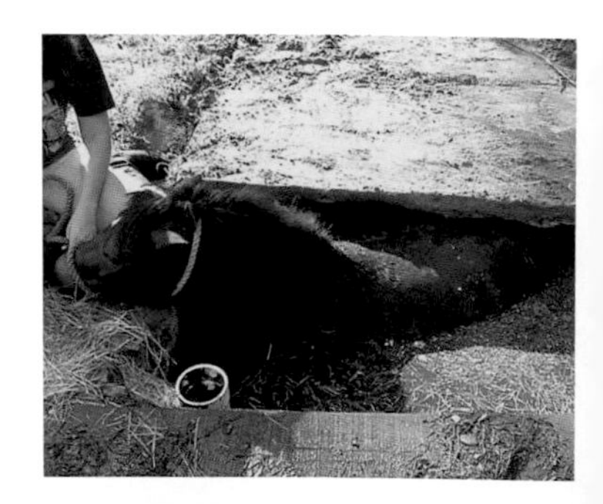

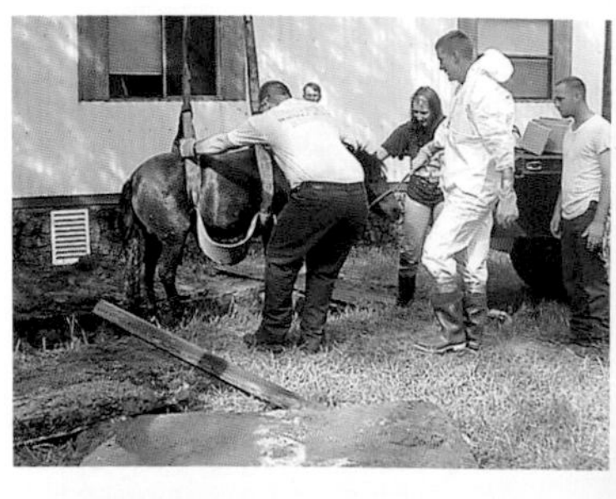

This story had a happy ending because the people took time to figure out their options and the pony was not in distress.

- Use plywood or boards to walk on mud. The horse can be rolled onto plywood and pulled over surface of mud (may need sedation for this).
- Put a blanket or space blanket on the horse to help him maintain body temperature, if in cool weather.
- Offer the horse water. Give him hay or grass to keep him calm, if he seems able to eat and he's not lying on his side and his head or neck position seem normal. Don't feed a horse that's in a septic tank.
- Flexible conduit can be used to thread a rope and then webbing under the horse (like a huge suture needle), since digging the mud is usually ineffective.
- Use webbing (or the saddle, if the horse is wearing one) around torso of body as an anchor point for haul. Be aware that the saddle may slip or pull free. Don't use winches to pull the horse, instead set up a rope system.
- Use forward assist or backwards drag (webbing around torso). Consider simple vertical web lift of animal.

Horse fallen through ice

- Determine if you can safely cut a three-foot-wide path through the ice and lead the animal out. Remove obstacles in the way of getting the horse out (trees, fence lines, etc.)
- Do not let anyone (even firefighters) approach the animal on the ice without surface ice rescue gear.
- Determine if the rescuer can safely halter the horse, and attach a long rope.
- Get an inflated inner tube for ice rescuers to put around the horse's neck and under his chin.
- Do not sedate the horse.
- Don't pull the horse out by the head. The lasso-and-pull method is not recommended except in extreme cases where the animal is drowning anyway.
- Allow surface ice rescuers to feed web around torso, if possible, to pull the horse out.

- Don't drag a horse across ice. Instead, pull the horse onto a tarp, board or gate, and drag the object with the animal on it.
- Get something to warm the hypothermic horse when he is removed (warm building, dry coat, blanket, etc.) and treat him for hypothermia as in Chapter 17, page 173 of this book.
- Get the horse's temperature, pulse and respiration, and provide first aid once it is out of the water.

Horse in a barn fire

- Call 911 or the fire department before you do anything. Call for help from friend, neighbor.
- Do not allow anyone to go into a burning building. People and horses can die from the roof collapsing on them. See if there's some way to get to the horses from the outside of the barn, a side door or knocking a hole in a wall.
- If a fire is caught early, have someone use a fire extinguisher at the base of the fire (Don't point it into the flames).
- Have someone catch, halter, and lead each horse individually from the outside door of the stalls to a paddock, round pen, or pasture.
- Horses should never be let out of a stall loose except as a last resort. In their frightened state they may run back into the barn to their deaths, or run out into the road to be hit by a responding fire truck.
- Do not attempt to recover anything (tack, valuables, etc.) from the barn.
- Obvious burn injuries should be treated as discussed in Chapter 6, page 57.
- Smoke inhalation is a less obvious and insidious injury and may damage the horse's lungs. Call the vet immediately if you suspect smoke inhalation.

APPENDIX

APPENDIX

GLOSSARY

Abscess: A pocket of infection located deep in the muscles or elsewhere in the body, surrounded by a thick wall of tissue.

Analgesic: Substance that controls pain.

Antihistamine: Class of drug that blocks allergic reactions.

Antibody: A protein produced by the immune system cells that attacks an infectious organism or other foreign substance in the body.

Antitoxin: An antibody against a toxin/poison produced by a bacterium.

Botulism: A type of food poisoning produced by the toxins secreted by the bacterium Clostridium botulinum, which causes progressive paralysis and usually death.

Caslick's Surgery: A common surgery performed on mares in which the lips of the vagina are sutured partially closed to prevent the entry of urine, manure or air.

Caudal: Facing the rear. A caudal splint would be on the "back" side of a leg.

Colic: Pain in the abdomen.

Contaminate: to allow infectious agents or foreign material (e.g., dirt) to enter the body, such as through a wound.

Cornea: The outer layer of the eye.

Dermatitis: Inflammation of the skin.

Dermatophilus: An organism that commonly infects the skin.

Edema: Swelling caused by accumulation of fluid in an inflamed area, by heart or kidney failure or following damage to the veins, arteries or lymphatic drainage system of an area.

Electrolyte: Salt that is normally present in the body and/or fed or injected to replace salts lost (e.g., sodium, potassium, chloride, bicarbonate).

Emphysema: disease of lungs characterized by an inability to completely empty out the air when breathing out.

Encephalomyelitis: Inflammation of brain and spinal cord.

Euthanasia: Humane destruction of the horse ("putting to sleep")

Expiration: Breathing out

Founder: Laminitis, inflammation of the sensitive/live tissues of the hoof.

Foreign: Not normally found in the body.

Hyperthermia: Body temperature above normal ("fever").

Hypothermia: Body temperature below normal.

Inspiration: Breathing in.

Intramuscular: Into a muscle.

Intravenous: Into a vein.

Jaundice: Yellow discoloration of the skin and mucus membranes (e.g., lining of the mouth) by pigments that accumulate in the body during liver failure or starvation.

Laceration: Rip/tear in the skin or other tissue (e.g., a tendon).

Laminitis: See "Founder."

Lateral: pertaining to one or both sides of something, such as a leg.

Membrane: An outer covering.

Mucus Membrane: Fluid-secreting linings of the mouth, nose throat, reproductive tract.

Myelitis: Spinal cord inflammation.

Narcolepsy: Disorder of the brain that causes an animal to appear to fall asleep inappropriately (e.g., while eating). A form of epilepsy.

Neoplasm: Abnormal growth, tumor.

Opthalmic/Opthalmologic: Pertaining to the eye.

Patent Urachus: Open connection between the urinary bladder and the umbilical cord in a newborn foal.

Pleuritis: Inflammation of the tissues lining the chest and covering the lungs (usually caused by infection).

Renal: Pertaining to the kidney.

Rhino/Rhinopneumonitis: A common respiratory viral infection in horses.

Salmonella: A common bacterial infection of the intestinal tract.

Sclera: The "white" of the eye.

Subcutaneous: Under the skin.

Tetanus: A rigid paralysis caused by toxins produced when a wound is infected with the organism Clostridium tetani.

Toxoid: A "tamed" version of a toxin that is injected into the animal to stimulate his immune system to product antibodies that will be ready to guard against that specific poison.

Toxin: A poisonous substance, harmful substance.

Tracheotomy: Making a hole in the trachea ("windpipe").

Tracheostomy: Inserting something into the trachea to keep a surgical opening open.

Ulcer: Any defect in the surface of a tissue, usually caused by surface tissues being injured and defective in some way.

IMPORTANT EMERGENCY INFORMATION FOR THE VETERINARIAN

- Horse's name:

- Age, breed, sex and use of the horse:

- Temperature, pulse and respiratory rate: (TPR) (See page 226.)

TIME	TEMP	PULSE	RESP
TIME	TEMP	PULSE	RESP
TIME	TEMP	PULSE	RESP
TIME	TEMP	PULSE	RESP

- Appetite and water consumption:

- Amount and any changes in manure:

- Nature of problem, if known. Symptoms and time:

- Has horse ever had this problem before?

WHEN

DIAGNOSIS THEN

TREATMENTS

RESPONSE TO TREATMENT

- When did symptoms start?
  Have they worsened, improved or remained the same?

  ____

  ____

- If bleeding, how much?

  ____

  ____

- Has horse received any treatment yet?

  ____

  ____

- Is the horse on any regular medications or has he been treated with any drugs or herbal supplements recently (including dewormers or tranquilizers)?

  ____

  ____

- Is the horse allergic or unusually sensitive to any medication?

  ____

  ____

- Any recent change in feed or environment?

  ____

  ____

- Other comments/observations:

  ________ ______________________
  TIME OBSERVATION

  ________ ______________________
  TIME OBSERVATION

  ________ ______________________
  TIME OBSERVATION

IN CASE OF INJURY

To put in the truck and the trailer in case you are injured.

Attention Fire/Rescue/EMS/Veterinarian

- My information:

MY NAME

ADDRESS

CITY, STATE, ZIP

PHONE (HOME) PHONE (CELL)

- Veterinary records, health certificates, Coggins tests for the horses in this trailer are:

GIVE LOCATION

- My insurance information for the horses in this trailer:

OR LOCATION

- Horse-familiar friend or family member authorized to make decisions about my horses, in case I am injured or incapacitated:

NAME

ADDRESS

CITY, STATE, ZIP

PHONE (HOME) PHONE (CELL)

- Alternate horse friends that can help transport my horses:

NAME

ADDRESS

CITY, STATE, ZIP

PHONE (HOME) PHONE (CELL)

- Insurance company for truck/trailer issues:

NAME: US RIDER, INC

PHONE

- My regular veterinarian(s) for these horses:

NAME

ADDRESS

CITY, STATE, ZIP

PHONE (WORK) PHONE (CELL)

Statement: "If my animals are injured or in need of care and I am unable to do so, please contact the closest local large animal veterinarian immediately. I authorize treatment of my animals by a licensed veterinarian. I authorize humane euthanasia in the event of a licensed veterinarian's recommendation."

SIGNED DATE

SIGNED DATE

You may have to get this notarized.

INDEX

A

B

C

D

E

F

G

T

U

V

W

X

Z

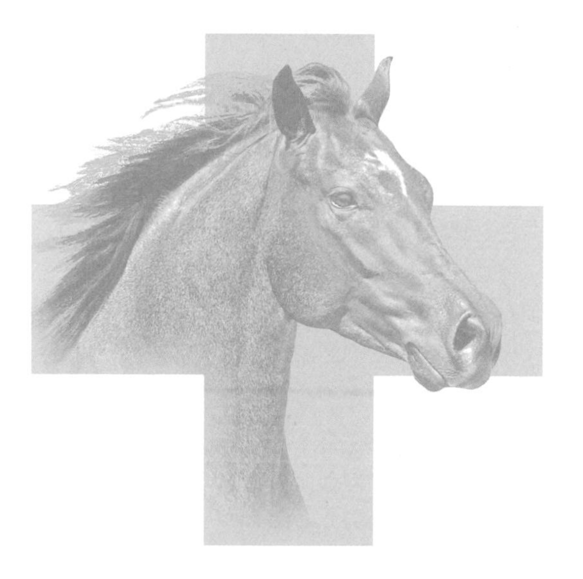

EMERGENCY PHONE NUMBERS

- Regular veterinarian

  ____

- Back-up veterinarian

  ____

- Full service veterinary hospital

  ____

- Horse owners

  ____

- Agricultural extension agent

  ____

- Poison control center

  ____

- Rescue Squad

  ____

- Vanning/Trailering service

  ____

- Fire company/Fire rescue

  ____

- Police: local

  ____

- Police: State

  ____

- Insurance company

  ____

- Neighbors and experienced horsemen

  ____